Praise for *Reclaiming Wellness*

"If you've ever wondered about the origins of the world's best lifestyle choices for the healthiest body and mind, this book is for you. Or if you are looking for ways to incorporate plant-based foods, spices, and herbs into nutritious, delicious meals, this book is for you. You'll find easy ways to keep your body and mind feeling fresh and vibrant, and you'll learn about your ancestors, too!" — **Jenné Claiborne**, chef and creator of Sweet Potato Soul

"In *Reclaiming Wellness*, Jovanka Ciares has brilliantly interwoven the power of multicultural ancestral traditions and wellness practices into a holistic road map to achieve optimized health even with the noise and chaos of the modern world trying to overwhelm us into dis-ease." — **Jason Goldberg**, author of *Prison Break*

"Jovanka Ciares is a miracle worker, a trusted source for wellness transformation from the inside out. Her wisdom and knowledge have healed and helped so many; may this book support you in reclaiming your wellness journey." — **Kelly Lynn Adams**, award-winning entrepreneur, business and life coach, and podcaster

"*Reclaiming Wellness* offers a fresh exploration of time- and science-proven popular wellness modalities. I truly enjoyed reading it. Jovanka Ciares uses the historical context of these practices to inspire you to get excited about trying and implementing them in fun, easy ways." — **Dr. Neeta Bhushan**, host of *The Brave Table* podcast, founder of Globalgrit.co, and cofounder of Dharma Coaching Institute

"I love everything Jovanka Ciares does. Her energy and knowledge of well-being are infectious. *Reclaiming Wellness* is a wonderful guide to understanding the root of many well-being practices and offers easy, fun, and useful ways for you to feel like your most radiant self." — **Tara Stiles**, founder of Strala Yoga and bestselling author of *Yoga Cures*

"*Reclaiming Wellness* is like discovering a hidden spring that refreshes you with long-lost secrets of balance, vitality, and well-being. Everything you need to get started is here — from the theory and the ancient history to guided exercises that steep you in the deep serenity, peace, and healing that are your birthright. Jovanka Ciares proves a gentle and expert guide, seamlessly combining personal stories and visualizations along with a comprehensive exploration of trusted ancient practices, structured schedules, and helpful resources. The result is a book that is simultaneously a joy to navigate and easy to use. *Reclaiming Wellness* is a gift from our own past; it offers the kind of compassionate and accessible guidance that awakens and encourages you to live each day fully alive, with enthusiasm and an open heart." – **Donald Altman, MA, LPC**, bestselling author of *The Mindfulness Toolbox*, *One-Minute Mindfulness*, and *Clearing Emotional Clutter*

"Jovanka Ciares is the real deal! She is a brilliant healer with a deep understanding of how to get to the root cause. Her book, *Reclaiming Wellness*, will provide you the blueprint to experience a full healing transformation with ease and grace. This is a must-read for anyone ready to reclaim their health on their terms." – **Dr. Mariza Snyder**, bestselling author of *The Essential Oils Hormone Solution*

"*Reclaiming Wellness* is the most inspiring and informative book on the true origins of modern wellness practices I've ever read. Jovanka Ciares masterfully weaves together empowering practices that even beginners can follow in order to massively improve their health and, therefore, their lives. Most importantly these powerful, ancient techniques have finally been framed within their correct historical context so that we can appreciate the diverse cultures and communities that paved the way for our collective ability to heal today. Thank you for this wonderful and important book, Jovanka!" – **Grace Smith**, hypnotherapist, *Wall Street Journal* bestselling author of *Close Your Eyes, Get Free*, and founder of GetGrace.com

"Jovanka Ciares brings us back to the heart of health and healing through culture, community, and history. Sometimes it feels difficult to know how to start or restart the healing journey. This book reminded me of the ways I am caring for my body and introduced me to so many easy things I can start doing right here and now. I've never before read a book that centers on the Black Latinx experience around health, healing, and history. The world needs more stories and practical ways to reclaim wellness, and Jovanka is leading the way." – **Ivelyse Andino**, CEO and founder of Radical Health

"Jovanka Ciares is the example we all should follow in reclaiming our wellness. Her healing journey began with gut health issues, which then led to her exploration of age-old wellness practices from many cultures. Her recipe for success is simple, yet she dives deep into the pillars of gut health that in turn set the foundation for total wellness. Her Reclaiming Wellness Method includes meditation, movement, a plant-based diet, nature, and community — all modalities key to leading people back to wellness. Read this book and find your path back to a healthy, happy life!" – **Vincent M. Pedre, MD**, functional medicine certified practitioner

Reclaiming
WELLNESS

Reclaiming
WELLNESS

ANCIENT WISDOM FOR
YOUR HEALTHY, HAPPY,
AND BEAUTIFUL LIFE

JOVANKA CIARES

Foreword by Julieanna Hever

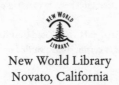

New World Library
Novato, California

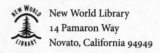

New World Library
14 Pamaron Way
Novato, California 94949

Text design by Tona Pearce Myers

Library of Congress Cataloging-in-Publication Data

Names: Ciares, Jovanka, author.
Title: Reclaiming wellness : ancient wisdom for your healthy, happy, and beautiful life / Jovanka Ciares.
Description: Novato, California : New World Library, [2022] | Includes bibliographical references and index. | Summary: "Presents a holistic concept of health that encompasses the physical, mental, emotional, and spiritual aspects of a person's being, with special emphasis on wellness practices pioneered by Indigenous cultures and people of color"-- Provided by publisher.
Identifiers: LCCN 2022000234 (print) | LCCN 2022000235 (ebook) | ISBN 9781608687848 (paperback) | ISBN 9781608687855 (epub)
Subjects: LCSH: Health. | Well-being. | Self-care, Health.
Classification: LCC RA776 .C54645 2022 (print) | LCC RA776 (ebook) | DDC 613--dc23/eng/20220127
LC record available at https://lccn.loc.gov/2022000234
LC ebook record available at https://lccn.loc.gov/2022000235

First printing, April 2022
ISBN 978-1-60868-784-8
Ebook ISBN 978-1-60868-785-5
Printed in Canada on 100% postconsumer-waste recycled paper

New World Library is proud to be a Gold Certified Environmentally Responsible Publisher. Publisher certification awarded by Green Press Initiative.

10   9   8   7   6   5   4   3   2   1

*To you, the reader and wellness seeker,
and to the healers of your ancestry, who live through you.*

Heal yourself, with beautiful love.
Always remember, you are the medicine.

— MARIA SABINA

Contents

Foreword

As it is for many, my journey toward finding an optimal diet has been quite curvy, with much nuanced information, accumulated wisdom, and ongoing investigation along the way. Eating plants piqued my curiosity after I read John Robbins's now-iconic book *Diet for a New America* as a teenager and found out how food actually ended up on the plate. This awareness disrupted my understanding of how the world worked and sparked the realization that my choices have a powerful impact not only on my health but also on those around me.

My early attempts at cutting out animal products were less than ideal. I had little wherewithal in the kitchen and limited access to information, as the internet was in its infancy and not accessible to the layperson yet. Thus, I scrambled to make my diet work by eating side dishes and snack foods. This process was interrupted by well-meaning and worried loved ones. My mom and dad, being concerned and caring parents, worried about me attaining adequate nutrition, so they enlisted our family friend, a nurse, to educate me on the real risk of my becoming deficient in certain nutrients by omitting animal products. We had this conversation over a teriyaki steak with a pineapple ring on top. I will never forget my first bite of that steak; fear of deficiency was driving me to comply, but once you know, you can't unknow.

Of course, I went back to eating the normalized, standard Western diet, but since I had not read any headlines of vegetarians dropping like flies, I knew there had to be more to this story, and my investigation continued. I was on a mission to get to the bottom of this and understand.

Years later, after I had accumulated a deep knowledge of medical nutrition therapy, biochemistry, and statistics and was able to dive directly into the scientific literature, everything made sense. I transitioned my diet successfully, experiencing extraordinary health benefits, and then applied what I had learned to my clients in my dietetics practice. With all this information and experience, I was able to build a thriving practice as a registered dietitian, author, lecturer, and podcaster that centers on plant-based living and mindfulness, with the goal of making evidence-based nutrition information accessible and simple to consume.

There is too much complexity today when it comes to nutrition. Everybody eats; therefore, everybody feels they are an expert on what we should and shouldn't eat. The resulting information overload is confusing for the layperson, who is simply trying to understand and implement a healthy diet, as well as for the researcher or healthcare professional, who struggles to communicate or interpret the data because it's so varied and often conflicting. My twenty-five-plus years in the health and fitness industry have taught me that finding the right approach to healthy living and wellness should be easy and intuitive. Seek out the habits that serve you and your goals best, focus on wholesome plant foods, and keep it simple. This is the approach Jovanka Ciares lays out so beautifully, holistically, and cleverly in *Reclaiming Wellness*.

When I was executive director of EarthSave International, I worked with a food bank located in a food desert in Sacramento, California, where we helped participants learn how to eat healthfully on a budget. The results were phenomenal, as expected. When you change your diet and lifestyle, your health improves. I love to say that results *are* typical. This type of work is hugely important, and I am grateful that many are focusing on it in underserved communities around the globe. Of course, there is always so much more that can and should be done. We can help create and/or expand community gardening projects, healthy living education, and access to wellness practices as a whole.

With that said, in order to get results, a person must be ready to change. As my father recently said to me after he suffered from a stroke, "Jule, you have to want it." Oftentimes people reach that point of readiness for change after watching an inspiring film, reading a book, or seeing a loved one suffer through a difficult diagnosis or even die. They have to arrive at the point where they are ready.

I believe *Reclaiming Wellness* can be that inspirational read that leads many people to make decisions that will ameliorate their health. The book is full of great suggestions and areas of wellness to start with, and I expect it to resonate with a lot of people.

Jovanka lists a wide variety of options in the book, and there is truly something for everyone, regardless of where they are on their healthy living journey. As you read through it, find the ones that resonate with you the most and explore them without any obligation to commit to them. It's just like when you're transitioning to a plant-based diet: you just try a new ingredient or a new recipe that you have never tried before, and if you love it, great — add it to the repertoire. If you don't, modify it or don't ever make it again, and move on. There are infinite tasty combinations of vegetables, fruits, whole grains, legumes, mushrooms, nuts, seeds, herbs, and spices to enjoy and thrive on. All you have to do is optimistically explore these practices and have fun.

— JULIEANNA HEVER, MS, RD, CPT, Plant-Based Dietitian®,
author of *The Choose You Now Diet* and
Plant-Based Nutrition (Idiot's Guides)

Introduction

Wellness is this amazing, seemingly elusive state of being that as a young adult I struggled to attain. That is, until my body decided to rebel and gave me what I once called a "smackdown" in the form of various chronic diseases — though thankfully, none life-threatening. Back then, I had no choice but to find alternative solutions to my health issues, and I embarked on an over-fifteen-year journey that changed my life for good. But wellness is not meant to be something we reach for only when we're in pain; it is not meant to be something we push for only after a diagnosis. Wellness is something we work for and achieve with daily practices, choices, and behaviors.

Today, this very moment, is the perfect time to talk about you and how you can become well. It is the perfect time to talk about whole foods, herbal remedies, and other wellness practices. Some of these may seem inaccessible, but all are within reach once we know how and, most importantly, why they work.

Growing up in Puerto Rico, I didn't see a lot of the preventable diseases that are common in the modern era. My mother's parents would be considered obese by today's standards, but they were otherwise healthy and didn't need medication or treatments until their late seventies and eighties. We had a few neighbors who might also have been considered unhealthy, but so few that you could have counted them with both hands and had a few fingers to spare. We rarely ate in fast-food restaurants. In fact, in my early childhood, there was only one fast-food restaurant (a KFC) in the area, and by the time I became a teenager, there was a second one (a Burger King). We ate homemade foods, rarely from a can — yes, even our beans were soaked and slow cooked — and definitely no soda. The biggest sources of sugar came from fresh fruit from the local market or the neighbors' yards, and our "junk" food was mostly fritters made at home with some natural ingredients. We were a group of healthy, laid-back, uncomplicated island people, thriving with very few resources and even less stress. Wellness was within me; it was part of my DNA, part of my upbringing. Today, many of these practices from my heritage are what I use to help myself stay well.

We don't have to move to a tropical island and eat fruit from a neighbor's mango tree to attain wellness. Some of the most effective practices to help become healthier and happier are not only within reach but within us. They are the practices our ancestors perfected and passed on from generation to generation. These include some of the most popular activities in the wellness world, ones that are embraced by billions of people who spend over $52 billion a year in the United States alone. And they can be reclaimed by you, without breaking the bank, as part of your ancestry and your birthright. All you need is the curiosity to learn from the past, a little planning, and a jolt of motivation.

1

Wellness: It's Not Just for the Privileged Few

How many times have you read an article or picked up a brochure at the health clinic reminding you of the plethora of health issues you are predisposed to because of your age, gender, or ethnicity? If you are a woman of color like me, then chances are, it's too many times to count. From chronic conditions like IBS, endometriosis, and eczema to life-threatening ones like heart disease and type 2 diabetes, aging seems filled with doom-and-gloom scenarios, especially for people of color and women.

Thankfully, it doesn't have to be. Every day, more and more people embrace lifestyle changes and practices to improve their health and well-being. They are actively pursuing activities that will inspire them to participate more each day in the world of wellness, rather than waiting for the wellness industry to invite them in. This book is dedicated to showing you how to do the same, no matter your age, gender, ethnicity, income, or social status.

The modern wellness industry has a diversity and inclusion

problem. The lack of representation within the wellness industry is palpable, from practitioners and advocates to brands that seemingly cater to only one type of audience — wealthy, white Westerners. In fact, you could be forgiven if you thought that some of the most popular modern wellness practices today, like yoga or meditation, were created by new age, Silicon Valley types in the last few decades solely for the benefit of well-to-do spiritual seekers and health advocates like themselves. Nothing could be further from the truth. Wellness is not for the privileged few. Wellness is a state of living that applies to all living creatures — humans, animals, and plants. And the most popular wellness practices have been practiced for millennia by people all over the world. Wellness is a way of life that emerges from and is for all of us.

This includes things like the growing popularity of a plant-based diet, meditation, and using saunas and hot springs to improve health. In fact, many modern wellness practices were first embraced by the poorest members of society before they were embraced by the elite (which I discuss more later). Thanks to these people, their discoveries, and their passion to pass on what they learned to each generation, we enjoy and benefit from these practices today.

To me, *wellness* is an inclusive term that describes an individual's overall health and covers all aspects of one's being — body, mind, and spirit. Working to attain a state of wellness involves long-term changes to our entire lifestyle, not just focusing on only one aspect of life. The goal of this book is to enhance your entire self, including your emotional, physical, mental, spiritual, social, and environmental well-being.

For instance, let's say someone wants to lose twenty pounds. Achieving that specific physical goal in a lasting, holistic way would include learning which foods nourish their particular body best. They would explore how different foods interact with one another as they travel through the body, impacting digestion, energy, and long-term health. They would also learn about how the foods they enjoy are made and produced, making decisions based on the true environmental and social cost in terms of the resources, land, energy, and people needed to grow and produce the food. With this knowledge, the person will lose twenty pounds, for sure, while gaining the wisdom to make healthier, more responsible choices that improve their life in many mutually supportive ways.

Many years ago, my journey through wellness began in a similar way. I was almost twenty-five years old and had just moved to New York City, and I was eager to embrace all the amazing experiences that my new life had to offer. I was fit, flexible, and super cute. To others, I must have seemed the picture of health. But I was in pain almost daily. Like most college students, my finances were very limited, and I didn't pay much attention to what I ate. Most days, I survived on dried cereal for breakfast, a fast-food combo meal for lunch, and a chocolate candy bar for dinner. As you can imagine, this food provided no nutrients to support my body, and I had no knowledge of the consequences of such a dangerous diet. Despite my high-sugar, highly processed diet, I was so undernourished and stressed out that I ended up losing fifteen pounds — which I didn't have to lose — and I had regular digestive symptoms, from constipation and diarrhea to gas and bloating. These were so severe I would topple over and writhe in pain almost every night.

Eventually, my health issues "smacked" me into changing my behaviors. I made the decision to learn how to cook, and I developed a weekly routine of grocery shopping. Even though I grew up in a family that embraced home-cooked meals daily, and my mom and grandma taught me basic cooking skills, I hadn't bothered to cook or shop on my own until that moment.

The process of learning how to make different dishes taught me valuable lessons about nourishing and honoring my body as the amazing machine that it is. This wonderful, imperfect body allows me to live, thrive, feel, ache, care, and love, and it deserves to be cared for the best way I know how. I am immensely grateful that I had youth and time on my side as I embarked on this journey of learning how to do that. I did not have a life-threatening disease, and I could make lifestyle changes relatively easily. But no matter what our personal circumstances, we are never powerless. There is so much we can do to support our body and restore balance and a sense of peace, to get as close to homeostasis — or a state of health and well-being — as possible. My hope is that this book will help you create that for yourself, regardless of your skin color, nationality, race, ethnicity, or socioeconomic circumstances.

Thankfully, more and more multicultural communities in the West are actively creating space for and embracing wellness practices. They are no longer waiting to be invited to the party. Wellness arises from all of us and it's meant to benefit all of us.

Whether you are new to wellness or various specific practices or not, I hope this book provides you with the knowledge to create your own wellness journey. Without knowledge, we can be at the mercy of others — like advertisers and wellness gurus — who want our business and have their own agendas. Some would have us believe that only certain brands or expensive programs can foster wellness. Instead, I encourage you to explore and to question, to increase your knowledge and to trust yourself, as you evaluate what practices might be best for you and which might be inappropriate, unhelpful, or even dangerous. Be curious about what could lead to a healthier, stronger, happier version of you, and pursue that curiosity to create just that.

The Big Picture: Wellness Is Holistic

Wellness is for everyone: young and old, sick and healthy, rich and poor, and all races and ethnicities. Wellness also includes everything, or all aspects of our lives, and the ultimate goal is to achieve positive, sustainable, long-lasting changes. Wellness is not a single thing we do, it doesn't happen all at once, and our wellness practices should increase happiness, not feel like a chore.

Ideally, wellness is how we unlock and access the full potential lying within. This isn't about following lifestyle rules to a T, but rather understanding our choices and owning them. We will certainly encounter roadblocks during this process, and that's to be expected! Pursuing wellness with an "all-or-nothing" attitude is a nonstop ticket to frustration and failure. Instead, if we accept ourselves, and trust the natural process, things will slowly fall into place. Wellness is about creating balance and strengthening the connection between our physical, mental, and spiritual selves. As a result, what we do to achieve wellness will vary depending on what needs more attention at any particular time. For instance, if our spiritual life is strong but our physical activity isn't, then we might find balance by focusing more on our physical self, while continuing to strengthen all the other parts that make us who we are.

In the big picture, wellness is about being at peace in and with the world. We are each an integral part of the whole that we call the universe. The energy that emanates from each of us, as well as from plants and animals, is interconnected. Our daily choices touch millions of lives, whether we realize it or not. Being aware of this interconnectedness fosters a holistic awareness of our place in the world and helps us make positive, conscious choices every day in our lives.

Health in the United States Today

The United States is the wealthiest nation in the world, and it knows how to spend! Americans spend more on healthcare per person than any other country, yet the nation consistently ranks lowest in comparative health-care outcomes. I've often wondered why we worry so much about terrorism and natural disasters when the standard American diet is what we should fear the most:

- In the United States, approximately 33 percent of adults are overweight, another 38 percent are obese, and 8 percent are extremely obese.
- Heart disease, stroke, and cancer — diseases affected by diet and lifestyle — account for over 50 percent of all deaths in the United States each year.
- Nearly half (47 percent) of American adults have high blood pressure, a precursor of heart disease.
- About 38 percent of Americans have high cholesterol, a major cause of heart attack and stroke.
- About 80 percent of heart disease–related deaths can be prevented with diet and lifestyle choices.
- In America, 50 million people have at least one autoimmune disorder that reduces their quality of life.
- The United States has one of the lowest life expectancies in the industrialized world.

Reclaiming Wellness: Own Your History, Own Your Health

Some of today's most popular wellness practices can trace their history to parts of the world and cultures historically populated by people of color. Every society has pursued wellness, and as a woman of color living in the United States, one of my goals is to share this multicultural history and to encourage all people, but especially people of color, to embrace the knowledge and wisdom of their particular ancestry and heritage. To me, owning your history is a part of owning your health and creating your own personal wellness journey. Yoga, for example, is now a very popular and widespread wellness practice, yet it's one of the world's oldest physical disciplines, having been developed in northern India over five thousand years ago.

Meanwhile, the use of plants as medicine — that is, herbalism and the use of modern supplements — has been part of every culture and every ethnic group since the beginning of time. In South America, shamans have been helping people heal using medicinal plants since precolonial times. Similarly, most ancient cultures developed their own plant-based diets to foster good health, diets that emphasized mostly local plants, grains, nuts, and seeds, while consuming expensive animal flesh only in small amounts and on special occasions.

Today, the wellness community invites people to incorporate ingredients from all cultures into their daily diets, sometimes touting them as "superfoods." Yet I believe that learning the history of these foods and their health benefits can excite you to embrace them. In in-person workshops, I include popular herbal blends and ingredients with medicinal properties, making sure to explain the places these amazing ingredients come from, honoring the land and the people who carried their knowledge from generation to generation. If the workshop is about stress management, for example, I often incorporate adaptogenic botanicals indigenous to every corner of the world to emphasize how almost every culture has had amazing products and practices that we can still use today: maca from the Andes Mountains in South America, ashwagandha from the dry regions of India and Africa, and aloe vera from the Arabian Peninsula. This inclusivity is a powerful educational tool. It reminds us that these foods are part of our shared human legacy, our DNA, whatever our personal background or culture.

I want every single person to know that their culture has played a role in the wellness practices that have become popular in the West. These practices are truly amazing at helping us restore and maintain health, and using them is part of how we honor the legacy of those who came before us.

Seven Wellness Concepts

As a certified wellness coach and lecturer, I've identified seven wellness concepts or areas that are the most popular or impactful in the modern wellness industry. Curiously, these seven concepts all have one thing in common: They were originally created, developed, used, taught, and shared by a deeply diverse group of people from around the world. In my experience, these seven are also the easiest to implement regardless of someone's socioeconomic background or access to resources. Yes, people can spend thousands of dollars and lots of time pursuing each one, but none require expensive investments of time or money. Most are free, and all can be incorporated into anyone's existing daily routine.

Here are the seven practices (described in the next seven chapters) that make up the heart of this book:

1. Plants That Help Us Heal

The use of plants as traditional medicine is widespread in history, though cultural traditions vary and have different names. They include Ayurveda (India), traditional Chinese medicine (China), Kampo (Japan), shamanism (South America), and Western herbalism (Europe and North America). Every group of people around the world has benefited from the use of plants to address ailments and help the body heal. In today's world, the use of botanicals and other plants as supplements has become a multibillion-dollar industry, but I promise you, you don't need a ton of money to use them. As I share some of the history of this ancient practice, I hope you will feel confident to incorporate them into your daily wellness routine.

2. Going Within

Meditation, mindfulness, visualization, and contemplative practices help us connect our physical and emotional sides. These practices don't require any spiritual beliefs, and they aren't meant to replace someone's religion. They are like "mental workouts" that calm our bodies and our minds and instill peace. We can use them effectively to enrich our understanding of what is sacred and miraculous within.

3. Yoga and Other Forms of Movement

Movement is an integral part of wellness. While there are a number of movement-related practices, and all are helpful, I focus mostly on learning, using, and reclaiming yoga, as its popularity and benefits deserve special attention. In addition, yoga is the quintessential example of a popular wellness practice developed by people of color in ancient times that is now embraced by all regardless of age, health, or circumstance.

4. A Plant-Based Diet

Some wellness experts like to say, and with good reason, that improving our health is "80 percent about nutrition, 20 percent about everything else." Just like how putting crappy oil in a luxury car can reduce the car's performance and longevity, what we feed our bodies can impact our ability to stay healthy and to heal after illness. Modern data supports the dietary practices of our ancestors, which emphasized a whole-food, plant-based diet. This doesn't mean becoming a full-on vegan (unless you're ready), but it does mean adjusting the balance of our diet to include more health-promoting plants and less meat and processed foods. As the ancients understood, our wellness depends on what we eat.

5. Oil, Water, and Heat

For centuries, people around the world have used some combination of water, oil, and heat to help foster wellness — from saunas, steam baths, and sweat lodges to hot oil and Swedish massage. These are, to me, some of the funnest wellness practices because they not only promote healing but restore our mind and soul as well. Many cultures around the world have used these basic ingredients to promote wellness, and you can embrace them, too.

6. Music and Community

Social wellness is a vital part of achieving a state of well-being. And what better way to engage in a loving way with our community than with sound and music? Cultures around the world have long used sound and music as an integral part of the healing process. Meanwhile, all types of community contribute to wellness. Community is a critical ingredient without which we can never be whole and well.

7. Grounding and Nature

"Remember you are dust, and to dust you shall return." The concept behind this popular biblical quote (from Genesis 3:19) predates the Bible, and it is corroborated by modern science. We are part of the earth and the earth is part of us. Embracing practices that help us reconnect with nature and that protect and honor Mother Earth can help improve our health. The seventh wellness

practice reminds us that we are not far removed from our ancestors and that we are an integral part of all life. By fostering, in
simple ways, our connection to nature, we reclaim our rightful
state of wellness.

The Key to Success Is Preparation

I remember when I went out on my first real date as a teenager. I
was so anxious and eager for it to go well that I spent hours preparing and anticipating every detail of the outing: my outfit, my
hair, my mannerisms, even my smile. I rehearsed conversations,
coming up with dozens of potential scenarios and practicing an-
ecdotes in my head to make sure I sounded smart, witty, cute,
funny, sexy. Maybe you had a similar experience! I got advice
from my friends, who coached me on how to behave, what to say,
what not to do. Developing a new wellness lifestyle can be just
like anticipating that first fancy date. We have to prepare for the
known and the unknown to ensure that we are as successful as we
want to be.

Typically, pursuing wellness means changing bad or unhealthy habits and replacing them with better, healthier ones. I
know from experience how challenging this can be. Change always seems daunting, but it doesn't have to be. In fact, our bodies
are used to change: We are basically a new human, with new skin,
bones, hair, and cells, every few weeks. The rotation of the earth
and its orbit around the sun ensure that our environment is constantly changing — daily, monthly, quarterly, annually. Change is
as much a part of us as the air we breathe. If we embrace change
as a positive, it can become as easy as the passing clouds in the
sky. That said, when changing habits, it helps to prepare and make
changes slowly. In this book, chapters 2 through 8 include lots
of specific tips on how to reclaim these seven wellness practices.

Meanwhile, chapter 9, "The Reclaiming Wellness Method," explains how to prepare and plan for adopting all the healthier lifestyle changes you want to make. It describes a step-by-step process that isn't overwhelming. In addition, chapter 10, "Recipe for Success," is a twenty-one-day wellness plan that fully incorporates the seven concepts in a flexible, easy-to-follow guide.

Preparation is the key to success. I can't stress this enough. No one succeeds in a goal without some form of planning — and in some cases, like a first date, quite a bit of planning. Often when we start something new, we are excited and eager for the experience. We imagine success: charming our date or getting into better shape with revitalized energy. But will our initial excitement, our good intentions, be enough to sustain us along the bumpy road ahead? Do we know what we really want? Do we know what our goals are? Do we know why we're doing what we're doing? Are we emotionally ready for change?

This book will help you answer these questions about your wellness journey. Hopefully, it will make you excited and curious — like a teenager with a crush — about all the wonderful possibilities that await, and it will help you prepare successfully to achieve them.

So, are you ready?! Let's get after it!

2

Plants That Help Us Heal

Healing plants is my absolute favorite topic these days. I have been studying herbalism for almost two decades and incorporating it into my wellness coaching practice since 2013. Soon after moving to New York and being exposed to the cold weather, I embraced hot teas as a way to stay warm and grounded. Then I started to realize that the teas also helped settle my ever-achy stomach and were a fantastic way to reduce my dependence on sugary drinks. Looking for new teas, botanicals, and herbal blends, I explored neighborhoods across New York City, from Astoria to Chinatown, from Jackson Heights to Washington Heights. That was one of the most fun ways to learn about my new city and its dozens of ethnic enclaves. Also, as I visited local bodegas and markets, I learned about different cultures, the history of the plants I found, and of course discovered amazing foods. That was how my love affair with herbalism started, and my love continues to grow stronger with each new plant I learn about.

One of the main reasons why I love herbalism so much is because the use of plants as medicine is so ubiquitous. Most people practice or experience it, even without realizing they are. Cooking with parsley, rosemary, and other culinary spices is a form of herbalism. Steeping a tea bag in hot or cold water and drinking that infusion is practicing herbalism. Of course, those are the simplest forms of the practice. You need to be well-trained to safely use many other botanicals, but there are still quite a few available in local markets that anyone can use daily in a safe way. In this chapter, I've only included botanicals that have been well researched and have great safety data behind them.

But first, here's a brief history of herbalism itself.

A Brief History of Herbalism

The use of plants as medicine is as old as humans themselves. From ancient history to today's modern prescription drugs, we continue to rely on the power of plants to help make us whole. While many evidence-based pharmaceutical drugs are derived from medicinal plants, people around the world still use traditional herbal medicine in various forms. And today, more than ever, modern urban dwellers are embracing the wisdom of plants in their quest to address their health concerns in a more natural way.

Where does the practice of herbalism come from? It seems to have sprung up on its own within every ancient culture, rather than starting in one place and spreading to others. In every society, people became curious about their environment and experimented with the plants they found, documenting their findings and passing that knowledge from generation to generation.

In the Middle East and ancient Egypt, for example, tablets and papyrus document the use of thousands of plants, some of which we still use today: aloe vera, juniper, garlic, even cannabis. In India, the practice of Ayurveda documents the use of turmeric as far back as 4000 BCE.

Chinese medicine practitioners — who also developed acupuncture, among other alternative treatments — have been using hemp and reishi mushrooms since the Bronze Age. African healers, who were and are almost exclusively women, have been using coffee beans, shea "butter," and more than four thousand other local plants to keep their communities strong for thousands of years.

In Europe, medieval texts describe the use of herbs by monks and medical practitioners alike. In fact, a well-known folktale from Europe describes a group of thieves ransacking the homes of deathly ill people during the black plague. After they were apprehended, the judge wondered how they had remained immune to the highly contagious plague. The thieves admitted using a blend of concentrated oils — including cloves, cinnamon, rosemary, and other plants — and claimed that this strengthened their immunity and protected them from the plague.

In the Americas, Indigenous women also led the way, learning from the land and caring for their communities. The original peoples of Central and South America enjoyed the benefits of now-popular plants like maca, quinoa, and the beloved cacao (chocolate) for centuries before the arrival of the first Europeans. And we can thank the traditional herbal healers in North America for plants like chia and echinacea.

Over time, as people traveled and settled far away from their native lands, they brought these plants and their knowledge with them, and they also learned to incorporate the use of local botanicals. This led to the massive collection of *materia medica*, or the written collection of the medicinal uses of plants, that we still use to this day.

By the end of the nineteenth century and the development of modern medicine, we gained a greater understanding of the specific actions of these amazing plants, and today, modern research has corroborated the thousands of years of anecdotal evidence passed on from ancient healers.

In part due to lobbying by the powerful pharmaceutical industry, herbal medicine declined in popularity during much of the twentieth century, but in recent decades, it has gained in popularity once more. Herbalism is now recognized and accepted by both the medical community and the general population. In fact, the World Health Organization estimates that 70 to 80 percent of people around the world rely on herbal medicine for some or all of their healthcare. This includes not just developing nations but modern countries like Chile, Colombia, Germany, Sweden, and Japan, where doctors prescribe hundreds of herbal remedies to treat a variety of conditions.

If you've ever had chamomile tea, used shea butter on your skin, or enjoyed a hot cup of cocoa, you've practiced herbalism. Medicinal plants are everywhere and help us even without our knowledge. Even popular prescription drugs like morphine (poppy) and over-the-counter medicines like aspirin (willow bark) and throat lozenges (slippery elm) use botanicals as a primary ingredient.

Herbal remedies offer a unique set of benefits: They are safe, easy to use, and provide results in a relatively short amount of time.

Abuela Was Right

One of my fondest memories of Mami Eva — my *abuela* or grandmother — was of her in the kitchen cooking the most incredibly tasty dishes: Her Puerto Rican–style beans were legendary, her rice with chicken to die for, and her *asopaos* (thick stew-like soups) were rumored to wake up the dead. She was a rotund woman, with light brown skin and thick wavy hair, and her hugs could crush bones. Mami Eva had only a fourth-grade education: As the illegitimate child of an Afro-Latina with Taino blood and a red-headed, blue-eyed, freckled man whose family certainly didn't approve of or acknowledge my grandmother, she didn't have a lot of opportunities in life. She was pulled from school to go to work making homes for her wealthier, whiter relatives. She loved school, learning, and especially reading. When she realized she couldn't go back to school, she decided she would bring school to her. She devoured any books she could get her hands on and remained an avid reader for the rest of her life. She had a wisdom and knowledge that rivaled the most educated people I've known. She and my grandfather, Papi Jaime, would always say: "Books are the best teachers. They have all the patience in the world, never get frustrated, and will repeat the lesson over and over until you get it right."

Mami Eva was also a fantastic herbalist, even though she didn't quite refer to herself as one. She ran a de facto daycare center out of her home and sometimes had up to three babies or toddlers running all over the house. If a baby in her care was teething, she made a certain tea to soothe their pain. When we bumped our heads and got a huge swollen bump, she mixed things like butter and salt and applied it to the bump, making the swelling and pain go down in minutes. She blended ingredients like avocado, eggs, honey, and cinnamon to make hair protein packs, and she knew exactly what to give me to soothe my menstrual cramps. She had dozens of simple yet powerful remedies in her kitchen, or as I now call it, her *kitchen pharmacy*. My first exposure to things like oil salves, compresses, and other home remedies were at Mami Eva's home as she helped my sisters, cousins, and me enjoy healthy, happy childhoods with her foods, her plants, and her love.

Like Mami Eva, millions of elders all across the world have stories about remedies, plants, and foods they use to address ailments or simple symptoms. Before the advent of modern medicine, every family had to have some basic knowledge of native plants, such as which were beneficial or toxic and how to prepare and administer them as remedies. Historically, that knowledge and those remedies were developed by women, and both were passed down from mother to daughter, and from grandmother to grandchild.

Do you have similar childhood experiences with your own grandmother or great-grandmother? Do you remember an auntie who used natural remedies to treat basic ailments, even if she didn't call it alternative or herbal medicine? Whether someone considers using herbs and spices to be "medicine" doesn't make it less valid or effective. Even if you don't know such a person, I encourage you to ask the elders in your family if they have stories about using plants to heal. If asked, parents and grandparents might remember practices they've forgotten about. Record these precious stories, which are as important as family heirlooms, and the memories of these conversations can stay with you forever and empower you to one day pass on the knowledge to the next generation.

Ayurveda: The Science of Life

Ayurveda is a system of alternative medicine that originated from the Indian continent. It's believed to be over five thousand years old, the oldest healing methodology still in practice, and its ancient wisdom is still used by over 80 percent of people in India and Nepal and millions more in Southeast Asia. Because Ayurveda uses so many plants and food ingredients in its remedies and recipes, and because the modern wellness industry has embraced some of its products so fully, it deserves special mention when discussing herbal medicine.

Ayurveda sees health from a holistic point of view: Body, mind, and soul work together to maintain balance and promote a state of wellness, rather than reacting to and fighting disease. When our system is out of balance, diseases can develop that can be treated both by focusing on the body or system that needs healing and by rebalancing body, mind, and soul.

I have been learning and studying Ayurveda for almost a decade, and while I incorporate its principles into my wellness coaching practice, by no means do I consider myself an expert. You can spend decades studying this amazing healing methodology and still have a lifetime of learning to do. The main reason I love and use Ayurveda in my practice is twofold: First, it encourages us to learn the relationship between ourselves and the world and to use foods and botanicals to keep us healthy or help us restore our well-being; and second, it encourages us to learn about our own "blueprint" or constitution so we become better balanced individuals who then have better relationships with others.

To get an expert's perspective on Ayurveda for this book, I spoke to Rita Burgos of Rebuild Ayurveda, an Ayurvedic practice that specializes in emotional and nervous system challenges (such as addiction, anxiety, anger management, depression), digestive distress, and offering complementary support for other chronic challenges, such as autoimmune disorders, diabetes, thyroid conditions, and cancer.

Rita mentioned, "Ayurveda in itself is a compilation of thousands of years of a syncretic process of adaptation, but its core principles are about living in harmony with nature and understanding your true nature and spirit. And that, ultimately, we are spiritual beings and that we are trying to live in a way where the body is in a state of health."

The broader principle of Ayurveda is helping humans live in harmony with nature. To that end, Ayurveda uses food, herbs (lots and lots of herbs), and body therapies, but as Rita mentioned: "At its core, Ayurveda is about using the therapies to restore your own body's natural intelligence and wisdom. Herbs, body therapies, working with the digestion is all about teaching your body to know its inherent wisdom and its natural intelligence."

Rita had a wonderful analogy for how our mind, body, and soul influence one another to either help us stay healthy or become imbalanced. She said:

> In Ayurveda, we say that all disease starts from either what you eat with your body or with your mind. It could be a trauma, an undigested trauma from childhood that has evolved into becoming a disease because it was not fully "digested." In the same way, you could take in a food that was inappropriate for your body, and you do it over and over and over again, and then it becomes an undigested toxin in the body. Then this starts to create deeper layers of ill health and becomes more serious and relocates. So the first place to start is to pay special attention to what you eat and how you eat, but also how you experience life, and how you handle those experiences of life, both in terms of what kind of situations you put yourself in and what kind of equanimity you have in your mind to be able to properly move through those experiences. For example, say somebody is consistently overeating. You do it for a little while, for a short period of time, you don't have an effect. But you do it constantly over and over again, for weeks, months, and years, and that initial pattern of overeating becomes a pattern that continues to develop and build and becomes a chronic illness. The chronic illness could include obesity. It could include heart conditions.

Another example could be at the level of the mind. It could be overwork. Somebody just simply working like seventy hours a week. They don't stop working, and they are in a highly stressed state. That ends up relocating and becoming a whole other set of conditions that start to change their hormones, that start to change their cortisol levels. Why do they overwork themselves so much? How do we teach them to make better choices? How do we teach them more equanimity in their life? How do we teach them to draw boundaries and know that their version of 100 percent is to live a more rhythmic life with both work and breaks throughout?

Rita offered some amazing tips to help embrace the wisdom of Ayurveda in a holistic way:

- Start programs in your community that introduce young people to organic gardening, and plant medicinal herbs in those gardens.
- Educate young people about food access in their communities, about junk food versus healthy foods, and explain how our elders and ancestors ate.
- Teach people to cook.

As Rita says: "I understand that's really hard. Everybody is overworked and overstressed. It's even hard for me to teach my kids all of that sometimes because we are so busy. But those are the life skills that, as a community, we have to understand. Those are the basic fundamentals of learning how to be a healthy person — how to cook your own food in a healthy way, how to learn how to relax."

I couldn't agree with Rita more. We must learn how to nourish ourselves, how to see the act of cooking and feeding ourselves as the ultimate act of self-love. These things go hand in hand:

While cooking and feeding ourselves, we can also practice the art of nourishing our minds and souls.

About the Three Doshas

Ayurveda talks about three basic life forces or constitutions, known as doshas. Those are vata (space and air), pitta (fire and water), and kapha (water and earth). Every single person has a unique combination of these three doshas, making each and every one of us a specific, unique being, a universe within this universe. Often, one of these doshas is stronger than the others in some individuals. Also, depending on the time of year and personal circumstances, they can get out of balance. So, balancing these doshas is key to staying healthy.

Vata Dosha	Pitta Dosha	Kapha Dosha
Creative, imaginative, enthusiastic, energy in short bursts, quick learner, talkative	Sharp-minded, focused, orderly, competitive, passionate, confident	Easygoing, relaxed, affectionate, compassionate, loyal, stable, analytical
Dislike cold climates, worrisome, anxious, impulsive, jealous	Uncomfortable in hot weather, impatient, prone to tantrums, pushy, demanding	Stubborn, prone to depression, possessive, sluggish digestion, can feel stuck

Top (Legal) Herbs from Around the World

By distinguishing "legal" from "illegal" botanicals (see "A Few Words about Illegal Botanicals," pages 32–33), I am taking a humorous but still serious jab at society, which demonizes certain botanicals while embracing numerous pharmaceuticals and government-approved medicines that have well-documented dangerous, severe, and even life-altering side effects. Yes, many plants can cause harm, and some should be regulated and even restricted. But even potentially dangerous plants can have positive, therapeutic uses.

This section features a short list of those botanicals that are most popular, accessible, inexpensive, easy to use, and effective. There are many more plants that could be listed, and more potential uses and health benefits, but a complete list would be its own book (maybe next time). So remember, these are just a few of the botanicals that relate to each major world region to provide a taste of the amazing variety of plants at our disposal.

China and the Far East

- **Ashwagandha:** This relatively unknown herb is worth embracing. Also known as Indian ginseng, it reduces stress and mild anxiety, improves sleep, and can boost the immune system.
- **Cumin:** This herb is commonly used in many cuisines and is native to various parts of the world, but the spice is really popular in Asian countries. Cumin can relieve indigestion, reduce abdominal pain, and reduce IBS symptoms. It may also protect against cholesterol and heart disease.

- **Ginger:** This incredible root has powerful medicinal properties. Ginger helps with relieving pain and nausea, easing cold and flu symptoms, reducing inflammation, supporting digestion, reducing gas, and much more.
- **Gotu kola:** This is believed to have many health benefits, including enhancing memory and preventing dementia, promoting wound healing, and helping skin conditions. Gotu kola also has antidepressant and anti-inflammatory properties.
- **Reishi mushrooms:** Relatively new to people in the West, reishi is considered the king of mushrooms for its ability to enhance the immune system, reduce stress, improve sleep, and lessen fatigue. It is not a plant but a member of the awesome kingdom of fungi.

India and Southeast Asia

- **Turmeric:** The popularity of turmeric, the bright spice that gives Indian curries their yellowish color, has exploded in recent years and with good reason. Turmeric can improve digestion and reduce inflammation, and it has anticancer properties.

Middle East

- **Aloe vera:** Hailing from ancient Egypt and North Africa, aloe is widely used to treat a wide variety of skin conditions. Used internally, it can help relieve constipation and lower blood sugar levels, and it has antioxidant properties.
- **Castor oil:** Used in many cultures and brought to the Americas by enslaved peoples, this oil is a natural moisturizer

that promotes wound healing and fights skin conditions like acne and fungus. It can be taken internally as a laxative.

- **Frankincense:** High in anti-inflammatory effects, especially against arthritis, frankincense may improve oral health and gut function. Traditionally, it's used to reduce stress and anxiety and achieve high levels of spiritual connection.

- **Thyme:** This tiny but mighty spice is used to treat diarrhea, stomach aches, respiratory issues, persistent cough, and sore throats.

Africa

- **Rooibos:** A popular caffeine-free tea, rooibos is a native African plant that's rich in antioxidants, can protect the heart, and has been shown to help manage diabetes. There's also evidence that it can assist in weight-loss management.

- **Shea:** The butter we all love and use comes from the nut of the African shea tree. It is a great moisturizer, but it's also great at reducing inflammation, treats acne, and restores elasticity to the skin.

Europe

- **Arnica:** This is used topically to handle rheumatic pain, bruising, hematoma, contusions, and edema due to fracture. It also reduces inflammation and should always be included in any home first-aid kit.

- **Fennel:** With a strong reputation as a weight-loss aid, fennel is especially helpful for relieving indigestion, severe gas, and bloating, and it can reduce pain and inflammation in the GI tract.

- **Hawthorn:** The berries of this plant have been used as a heart tonic for hundreds of years. It improves oxygenation and pumping capacity and relaxes blood vessels. In Germany, it's used to help treat heart disease.

Central and South America

- **Cacao:** Known as the "food of Gods" and for good reason, this fermented product from cacao plant seeds can improve circulation, positively affect the mood and libido, and protect the heart. It is also a sweet delicious food. Enough said!
- **Cayenne pepper:** Considered one of the top "healers of the world," cayenne can improve circulation, stop excessive bleeding, and even help prevent heart attacks. It is antibacterial and antioxidant and also reduces pain and stiffness.
- **Maca:** A powerful adaptogenic root, maca is traditionally used to maintain stamina, boost energy, improve mood, and increase libido in both men and women. It is also known to help manage stress and reduce anxiety, and it may help relieve menopausal symptoms.

North America

- **Catnip:** Yes, the same herb beloved by your kitty is actually amazing for people. It is a digestive tonic that can help reduce gas and spasms. It has high antioxidant nutrients and phytochemicals that can help people sleep and alleviate headaches.

- **Elderberry:** This is a quintessential immunity builder and protector of respiratory issues related to the cold and flu. It also helps treat constipation, colic, diarrhea, sprains, and skin irritation.
- **Raspberry leaf:** A powerful tonic for the reproductive system, raspberry leaf can be taken by women in all stages of life: from first menses to menopause. It can be used to relieve cramps and pain and treat diarrhea, colds, and stomach complaints. It's even safe for pregnant women.

Reclaiming Herbalism: A Quick Guide to Botanicals

Of course, people don't use herbs based on what part of the world they originated from. We pick the plants to use based on our specific taste, needs, and goals, so here is a quick guide to how to use the botanicals described above. I've converted this information into a handy chart that you can copy and put on your wall or refrigerator door.

I highly encourage you to try all these botanicals for yourself. Research them further, see if they work for you, and if they do, use them regularly. The chart below includes the actions or known benefits for each botanical, the best way to use or consume them, and sometimes the typical dosage. Ideally, pick two or three botanicals that you're curious about and believe might be of benefit, try them for seven to ten days, and during that time, journal about how you feel after using them. Botanicals are fast-acting yet mild substances, so you probably won't notice a big jolt in your physiology. Rather, you should feel like something is supporting your system, like a loving hug from the inside out. All of these botanicals have helped me in more ways than one, and I think you will love them, too.

Botanical	Action (Benefits)	Form	How to Use
Aloe vera	Use topically for healing the skin; ingest capsules to relieve constipation, lower blood sugar levels, and for antioxidant properties	Topical gel and capsules	Use topically as much as needed; for capsules, take 25 mg a day with food
Arnica	For rheumatic pain, bruising, hematoma, contusions, edema due to fracture, and reducing inflammation	Topical gel	Use as often as needed
Ashwagandha	For reducing stress and mild anxiety, improving sleep, and boosting the immune system	Capsule or tincture	Take 300 mg twice a day
Cacao	For improving circulation, positively affecting the mood and libido, protecting the heart	Powder or food (chocolate)	Take or eat as needed
Castor oil	Use topically to promote wound healing, as anti-inflammatory, to protect hair and scalp; ingest as a laxative	Topical oil and capsules	Create a compress and apply oil to the area as needed; for capsules, take 25 mg a day with food
Catnip	For relaxation, boosting mood, reducing anxiety and nervousness, improving digestion	Dry leaves	Brew 2 tsp. per cup as a tea; 1–2 cups a day
Cayenne	For improving circulation, stopping excessive bleeding, and preventing a heart attack; reduces pain and stiffness	Powder	Dissolve 30 mg in a glass of hot water or hot cacao; use as spice in recipes

Botanical	Action (Benefits)	Form	How to Use
Cumin	For relieving indigestion, reducing abdominal pain, and IBS symptoms; protects against cholesterol and heart disease	Powder	Use as spice in recipes
Elderberry	For building immune system and treating respiratory issues related to cold and flu; treats constipation, colic, diarrhea, sprains, and skin irritation	Dry leaves	Brew 2 tsp. per cup as tea; 2–3 cups a day
Fennel	For aiding weight loss, relieving indigestion, severe gas and bloating, and reducing pain and inflammation in the GI tract	Seeds	Brew 2 tsp. per cup as tea; 2–3 cups a day
Frankincense	An anti-inflammatory, for improving gut function, asthma, oral health, and memory	Topical oil, usually an infused essential oil	Rub a couple of drops on your temple, back of neck, or in front of the elbow
Ginger	For relieving pain and nausea, easing cold and flu symptoms, reducing inflammation, supporting digestion, and reducing gas	Powder and root	Brew 3 inches of the root as tea; 2–3 cups a day; use powder as spice in recipes
Gotu kola	For boosting brain power, improving skin health, and promoting kidney and liver health	Capsule	Take 500 mg twice a day for 2 weeks, then pause for 2 weeks

Botanical	Action (Benefits)	Form	How to Use
Hawthorn	A heart tonic for improving oxygenation and pumping capacity and relaxing blood vessels	Capsule	300 mg daily
Maca	For improving memory, boosting energy and stamina, balancing hormones, and improving mood	Powder	Add ½ tsp. in a smoothie, oatmeal, or coffee drink
Raspberry leaf	For reproductive issues, such as relieving cramps and menstrual pain; also for treating diarrhea, cold symptoms, and stomach complaints	Dry leaves	Brew 2 tsp. per cup as tea; 2–3 cups a day
Reishi mushrooms	For enhancing the immune system, reducing stress, improving sleep, and lessening fatigue	Powder	Put ½ tsp. per cup in cold smoothie or hot coffee
Rooibos	An antioxidant for protecting the heart, managing diabetes, and weight loss	Dry leaves	Brew 2 tsp. per cup as tea; 2–3 cups a day
Shea	For reducing inflammation, treating acne, and restoring elasticity to the skin	Topical butter	Use as often as needed
Thyme	For treating diarrhea, stomach aches, respiratory issues, persistent cough, and sore throats	Dry leaves and fresh herbs	Consume 1 tbsp. of dried leaves twice a day; use as ingredient in recipes; infuse fresh herb in vinegars or raw honey for 2 weeks

Botanical	Action (Benefits)	Form	How to Use
Turmeric	For improving digestion and reducing inflammation; has anticancer properties	Powder and capsule Note: should always be combined with pepper	As capsule, take 1,500 mg a day; use as spice in recipes

Reclaiming Wellness Trivia

The Aztec Empire of Mexico and Central America used various herbs and plants for grooming and healing. They used the fruit of a tree called copalxocotl, which produced a lather used to wash their clothing and hair, and they used several plants to combat body odor and wore herbal-infused perfumes regularly. Their herbal healers treated everything from wounds and low-grade infections to broken bones with herbal blends and techniques, some of which were more effective than those known by the European colonizers at the time.

Most impressive, the Aztec's dental hygiene and treatment of diseases of the mouth using ingredients like geranium, charcoal, chili, and salt was so advanced that they rivaled some of today's dental practices. They even brought us the famous natural chewing gum (known as chicle) to freshen our breaths. Thank you, Aztecs!

A Few Words about Illegal Botanicals

As ancient cultures discovered, not all plants have healing properties. Some are poisonous or can be harmful if taken in high doses,
while other plants can do more than heal: They contain psychoactive chemicals that can affect consciousness, altering perception,
mood, and behavior. These entheogenic plants are not necessarily dangerous, but most are now illegal or are highly restricted
in modern society. For instance, plants like coca and poppy can
be turned into cocaine and opium, respectively, which are highly
addictive processed substances that can harm the body perma-
nently. Then again, poppy is also a key ingredient in morphine
and other prescription opioids used by the medical establishment
to manage pain. Psychoactive plants like cannabis (or marijuana)
and mushrooms that contain psilocybin also have mind-altering
properties that some doctors use to help ease pain for millions of
people annually.

Nevertheless, these drugs are so powerful that most governments around the world have made it illegal for individuals to
own, grow, distribute, or consume them, even when they are allowed to be prescribed by doctors for pain management. Cannabis
is a great example of this. Cannabis has been used since ancient
times by many societies; for instance, Napoleon's troops smoked
cannabis in lieu of drinking alcohol. Eventually, most countries
banned cannabis as a dangerous drug, though many people have
continued to use it illegally and advocate for it to be decriminal-
ized. They argue that, despite its mind-altering capabilities, it has
no proven dangerous actions and should be regulated by society
like alcohol.

Today, we know that cannabis has a proven capacity to relieve pain in patients with both chronic and life-threatening
conditions. As its use as medicine becomes more widespread, and
as millions experience its benefits, cannabis is becoming more

widely accepted and its use is increasingly being legalized. I've seen this shift in attitude in my own life: Even some of my conservative family members have opened their minds and hearts to the benefits of botanicals like cannabis, and my friends and clients tell me similar stories of loved ones reclaiming this wonderful plant.

There is still much to do. Governments, private citizens, and civic organizations must come together to continue to study and learn about the powerful medicinal properties of plants like cannabis and mushrooms with psilocybin. Then we must move to deregulate their use and reverse the damage caused by aggressive legal convictions for possession and distribution of cannabis, especially in communities of color. I hope that before long we can all experience the benefits of these plants safely and without fear of repercussion.

3

Going Within

I grew up in a conservative Catholic household, surrounded by a community who was very active in church-related activities. Growing up, my idea of meditation was something that hippies and flower children did, an activity that was in direct conflict with Christian dogmas; in other words, not something I should be concerned with at all. Prayer was encouraged instead. Sadly, it took until my midtwenties to realize that the practices of meditation and prayer are not in conflict with each other. On the contrary, they are highly complementary and can help strengthen our connection with our spiritual life.

When I was young, the prayers I was taught always left me feeling uninspired. It was almost like I was pleading, without any sense of empowerment as a cocreator of my own reality and the reality I was praying for.

Once I discovered meditation, a whole world of opportunities opened. With meditation I learned to listen to my intuition and the messages sent to me in a variety of ways by my guides, my ancestors, and the universe. I realized that I could dig deeper into the lessons the world was giving me and find a better connection with the spiritual world. This way, when it is time for prayer, it becomes more like opening up to a dear friend and mentor and asking for guidance, while letting go of the outcome, rather than a disconnected supplication to a force removed from me. In essence, I became a cocreator of my reality and my future.

This chapter describes how to embrace and develop a contemplative practice that connects you with your spiritual self regardless of religious beliefs. This includes meditation, visualization, and hypnosis, and exercises for all three appear at the end of the chapter. These practices are almost as old as humans themselves; they are part of our human ancestry, our DNA, and reclaiming them can bring a world of positivity into our lives.

Reclaiming Meditation

Meditation is a practice through which we achieve mental clarity and emotional stability. There are a variety of methods; many people meditate in silence and some use guided music and prompts. In the modern era, people practice meditation as a way to reduce stress, depressive feelings, anxiety, and pain and to enhance a peaceful state of mind.

Almost every culture around the world, at one point or another, has embraced meditative practices. The oldest documented evidence is from India: There is Indian wall art that dates to around 5000 BCE, and ancient Indian religious texts called the Vedas date to around 1500 BCE. However, all the world's major religions have incorporated the concepts of meditation into their practices.

Buddha is believed to have spread and popularized the practice in India. Taoism and Confucianism in China propagated meditation techniques in the Far East. Centuries later, Judaism, Christianity, and Islam all adopted contemplative practices to heighten spiritual experiences. In the twentieth century, hatha yoga and Transcendental Meditation gained worldwide popularity (for more on yoga, see chapter 4), in part thanks to the work of "self-help" gurus like Paramahansa Yogananda and Dr. Deepak Chopra, among many others.

In the second half of the twentieth century, meditation became very popular in the United States as students traveled east to study and train under meditation masters in places like India, Myanmar (Burma), Japan, China, and Thailand. Some became highly influential figures in the world of meditation and mindfulness, including Dr. Jon Kabat-Zinn, who founded the Mindfulness-Based Stress Reduction (MBSR) program in Massachusetts in 1979. His program uses mindfulness and meditation to help treat patients with chronic illness, and MBSR was instrumental in bringing attention to the health benefits of these practices.

Today, medical and scientific research includes hundreds of studies on meditation and mindfulness, including over two hundred randomized controlled trials from 2013 to 2015 alone. These confirm that meditation benefits both physical and mental/emotional conditions, including depression, anxiety, chronic pain, severe stress, and autoimmune disorders, among others.

Meditation is universal and can benefit anyone, regardless of religious or spiritual beliefs. Nor is there only one correct or effective way to meditate. There are dozens of different meditation techniques, and I encourage you to explore different options and find the ones you enjoy and that fit your lifestyle. Even meditating for just fifteen or twenty minutes is all you need to experience the benefits of this ancestral practice, which has helped billions of people for thousands of years.

Reclaiming Visualization

Visualization or guided imagery is a type of meditation practice in which we visualize in our mind a specific experience or outcome as if we were watching a movie. Many years ago, before it became more widely accepted, I was curious about it and wanted to explore how it might help me attain my wellness goals. Today, many people use it: Businesspeople use visualization to help achieve their work goals, athletes use visualization to help improve their physical performance, and everyday people use it to build a better life and a more positive attitude for themselves.

In the United States, visualization was popularized by alternative health advocates in the early 1980s. The modern methods are based on ancient Greek and Roman practices, and Shakti Gawain's 1978 book *Creative Visualization*, which has now sold over seven million copies, became one of the first and most popular reference guides. I read this book many years ago, and I still recommend it to my clients and students.

In her book, Gawain explains that creative visualization is the "art of using mental imagery and affirmation to produce positive changes in your life." Like meditation, the essence of visualization is simple, but many techniques and methods have been developed for using it. Again, I encourage you to explore these various systems, books, and courses, which aim to help people incorporate this technique into their contemplative practices.

I love the practice of visualization, but I also know that for many people who identify as BIPOC (Black, Indigenous, people of color), it can sound like some silly thing that Southern California hippies do. In fact, the tradition of visualization is deeply intertwined in the Indigenous cultures of nearly every region of the world, including the Americas, Africa, and Asia. Cultural traditions, history, customs, rituals, and legends were almost exclusively passed on through vivid narratives from the elderly to the young. Oral storytelling is a form of visualization, and each time a story was told, it brought the culture and its history to life, and it helped young people visualize their future in their imagination.

Indigenous peoples also used guided imagery (alongside smudging, drumming, and music) in their healing and religious practices. Of course, every culture had their own particular practices, which differed, but before the advent of writing, visualization and storytelling were how we educated ourselves and built dreams.

Today, we use visualization slightly differently, since we do not need to rely exclusively on oral storytelling to learn history. But we still have a similar goal of imagining what we want in our mind's eye as a way to help bring that vision to fruition in the real world.

Reclaiming Hypnosis

Maybe you're thinking: *Wait, did I read this right? Is she really talking about ... hypnosis?*

To which I would reply, yes, I am, though now the more commonly used term for this technique is *hypnotherapy*. I think it's vital for us to reclaim hypnosis because it offers amazing benefits, as it has for thousands of years.

Hypnosis has gotten a bad rap because of Hollywood's incessant and incorrect portrayal of it as a coercion technique, so let me start by explaining what hypnosis is not. No, hypnosis is not some magician on stage controlling someone's mind and making them dance against their will or cluck like a chicken. And no, if you've seen the movie *Get Out*, hypnosis is not some crazy rich white lady dragging your mind into a "sunken place" at the click of a spoon against a teacup and keeping your real self caged for all eternity (I love you, Jordan Peele, but, damn).

Hypnosis is, as my dear friend and world-renowned hypnotherapist Grace Smith explains, "meditation with a goal." If you've ever meditated or otherwise achieved a state of deep relaxation while still being aware of your surroundings and in control of your thoughts and body, you have experienced a type of hypnotic state. This is a real and powerful therapeutic tool with well-documented medical benefits.

During hypnotherapy, our eyes remain closed and we are guided to a state of deep relaxation, which is known as the theta brain wave state. This state is deeper and more relaxed than daydreaming and more conscious and alert than sleep. In this state our eyes are closed but we are awake, relaxed, and highly concentrated, focusing on a single idea or topic. In this deeply relaxed state, we can access our subconscious mind, which is in essence a data bank of information. According to Freud, the subconscious contains approximately 90 percent of our mental experiences: memories, emotions, dreams, beliefs, desires, values, and fears. Experts believe that all meaningful decisions are made at the subconscious level. If we, with the help of hypnosis, are able to change the information in this data bank to our advantage, we could then resolve issues that have been with us for years and for which other techniques have not been helpful.

According to the Mayo Clinic, hypnosis has been studied for multiple conditions, including the following:

- Pain management
- Stress and anxiety
- Symptoms of menopause, including hot flashes
- Behavioral issues like weight gain, smoking, insomnia, and cravings
- Reduction of symptoms in patients undergoing cancer treatment
- Other mental health conditions

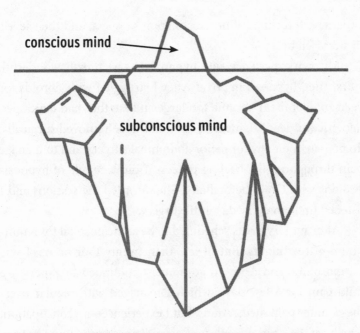

The conscious vs. subconscious mind

Dozens of studies have shown the efficacy of hypnotherapy to address various conditions. For instance, a 2018 *Time* magazine article entitled "Is Hypnosis Real? Here's What Science Says" states that in research conducted by Irving Kirsch at Harvard, study participants who received hypnotherapy in addition to CBT (cognitive behavior therapy) lost twice as much weight as those who only received CBT. The article continues, "Apart from aiding weight loss, there is 'substantial research evidence' that hypnosis can effectively reduce physical pain, says Len Milling, a clinical psychologist and professor of psychology at the University of Hartford."

Author of *Close Your Eyes, Get Free*, Grace Smith cites a study whose findings showed that "after listening to a hypnosis recording twice per day for only 7 days, participants experienced 32% more happiness [and] 58% less depressed feelings." They also experienced feelings of procrastination 51% less, and their levels of stress fell by 45%.

My own experience with hypnosis has been truly wonderful. I first tried hypnosis in 2014. After I struggled with fibroids for years, one of them became too large and another had developed necrotic (or dead) tissue, and they had to be removed surgically. To prepare mentally for major abdominal surgery and to manage pain throughout the healing process, I did a couple of hypnosis sessions with Grace beforehand. She recorded the sessions and I listened to them every day until surgery.

After surgery, I was scheduled to be at the hospital for a minimum of two nights. But in less than twenty-four hours, I was off morphine and ready to go home. I continued to experience mild pain for a few days, which I managed with regular over-the-counter pain medications, but I experienced no constipation, which can be a big side effect of general anesthesia. I was back in the yoga studio four weeks after major abdominal surgery.

A couple of years later, Grace helped me address a debilitating fear of flying. At the time I was living in Los Angeles and flew regularly to see my family in Puerto Rico. However, to handle the plane ride, I had to take strong antianxiety prescription drugs, which knocked me out for half a day. I once even missed a flight because the meds made me fall asleep at the airport while waiting to board.

This time, Grace and I did an extended two-hour hypnosis session, and I listened to a recording of that session every day for about a month. Ever since, I've been able to fly far and wide without anxiety or the aid of medication. Don't get me wrong — when there is heavy turbulence and the plane shakes in the air, I still get a big jolt in my chest. I'm still human, and hypnosis is not a magic pill that suddenly turns someone into a robot without any emotions. We wouldn't want that anyway! However, hypnosis removed the root causes of my fear and allowed me to release them so I can experience flying without anxiety. I can eat, watch movies, even do work while in transit without major issues. That's how powerful hypnosis has been for me.

The Ancient Roots of Hypnosis

The use of hypnotic states to promote healing has been part of almost every culture throughout time. According to Grace, hypnosis began in ancient Egypt, and not long after, it was used by the ancient Druids in what is now the British Isles. Later, evidence of hypnosis techniques appeared in Sumerian, Persian, Chinese, Indian, Nigerian, and Greek cultures.

One of the earliest references to hypnosis dates to the third century BCE. In ancient Egypt, the temple of Imhotep in the city of Saqqara was an important healing center where ailing people would journey in search of a cure from the gods. Various rituals included reciting rhythmic prayers and staying in a darkened chamber to induce a sleeplike state and allow the cure to be revealed. According to Grace, in these "dream temples," people were "encouraged to close their eyes and go into a dreamlike state while still awake, while priests and priestesses would speak 'magic words' into their ears, and the person would leave the temple having been forever transformed."

Later, hypnosis was one of the many ancient healing techniques that leaders of various Christian denominations, including Catholicism, tried to suppress and eliminate, vilifying them as "evil" and "against" Christian doctrine. In order to consolidate their power and control populations, church leaders did not want the masses to believe they could heal themselves on their own. For centuries, they pursued a systematic campaign to condemn all healing that did not involve ordained priests and subscribe to Christian or Catholic dogma and beliefs. The truth is, hypnotherapy in no way contradicts any aspects of Christian doctrine.

Thankfully, this art was not lost forever, and some people have always continued to use this practice to manage certain health issues. During World War I, when there was a shortage of anesthesia, doctors and nurses used hypnotherapy to decrease pain, while in cities at this time, dentists used it to manage teeth extractions and other treatments with relative success.

In the Americas, shamans and other Indigenous healers developed their own practices for inducing an altered state of consciousness. Some practices have included the use of mind-altering botanicals and extreme physical changes to facilitate healing, while others have used rhythmic drumming, singing, and dancing to cultivate a type of hypnotic trance in order to access the subconscious mind.

Since I agree with her completely, I will let Grace have the last word. Hypnosis is, she says, "one of the tools that multicultural communities could use to begin to heal subconscious ancestral trauma, so it is imperative that everyone have equal access to self-hypnosis education and that there is a mainstream understanding this tool exists and can be utilized by everyone effectively."

Practices for Reclaiming Meditation, Visualization, and Hypnosis

Here are four practices for reclaiming the techniques described in this chapter. Of course, there are dozens of variations for each, but these are good ones to start with, especially if you're new to these practices. Try each one for a week or so, and if it doesn't work for you, experiment with others. When I first started meditating, a dear friend recommended a meditation CD — back when CDs were still a thing — but that proved too cumbersome for me. I was too new to the process, and I found it very hard to sit quietly and still for more than three to four minutes.

Rather than judging myself too harshly, I talked to a friend, an experienced meditator, and he assured me that there is no such thing as a good or bad way to meditate. Instead, the goal is to find the style and type that works best for you, adapt it to your lifestyle, and make it your own. In the end, the most important thing is that you learn to tap into and produce a deep state of relaxation, a calm mind, and a nourished soul.

To start, here are two basic meditation exercises. One is a guided meditation that can be done while sitting or lying still, and the other is a moving meditation. The easiest way to do them on your own is to record the instructions so you can play them back and listen (rather than having to read along). Record yourself, or ask a trusted friend to read, on a computer or use your phone's voice memo function. Read slightly slower than your normal speaking pace.

GUIDED MINDFULNESS MEDITATION EXERCISE

This is a good start for people who prefer a little guidance or find it hard to sit quietly. In this exercise, the goal is to observe your wandering mind without judgment. When your mind starts to drift, simply let the thought go without attachment, and return to the prompts guiding you through your meditative journey.

To start, find a comfortable, quiet place, and either sit or lie down, making sure that your back and feet are supported and that you can let each part of your body fully relax.

- Take a deep breath, letting go of tension, and soften your jaw and shoulders.
- Take another deep breath. Breathe in for a count of four, hold for a count of five, and exhale for a count of six.

- Repeat this breath. Inhale for a count of four, hold for a count of five, and exhale for a count of six.
- Return to breathing normally, and scan your body for any signs of tension.
- Breathe in and notice the crown of your head and your forehead. As you breathe out, let any tension go.
- As you breathe in, notice your nose, your cheeks, your mouth, your lips. As you breathe out, let any tension in these areas go.
- As you breathe in, notice your jaw, your bite, your neck. As you breathe out, let that go.
- As you breathe in, notice your shoulders, your upper back, your chest. As you breathe out, let that go.
- As you breathe in, scan your arms, your elbows, your wrists, your hands. As you breathe out, let them lovingly relax.
- As you breathe in, notice your middle and lower belly. Are you holding them in? As you breathe out, let them relax.
- As you breathe in, notice your hips, your crotch, your buttocks. As you breathe out, let them lovingly relax.
- As you breathe in, scan your thighs, your knees, your calves. As you breathe out, let them relax.
- As you breathe in, notice your ankles, your feet, your toes. As you breathe out, let any tension go.
- Take one more deep breath in and scan your full body for any remaining tension. As you breathe out, let that energy flow away.
- Next, imagine a tiny bubble of your favorite color flowing toward you. Let that bubble sit a few inches from your head.

- As you breathe in, see the bubble fill up and get bigger and bigger. The bubble is filling up with protective, all-loving flow. As you breathe out, the bubble remains as it is.
- Take another deep breath in, and see the bubble fill till it is about to burst. As you breathe out, let the bubble burst. Out of it comes a sweet, soft wave of protective, all-loving energy that covers every inch of your body, starting at the crown of your head and moving down, down, down, until it covers your toes.
- This energy is your energy. It is now back where it rightly belongs, supporting you, replenishing you, and filling you up.
- Stay with that energy as you take a final deep, long, letting-go breath. Thank yourself for allowing this practice today.
- Stay in this position for as long as you need to. When you're ready, open your eyes and continue with the rest of your day.

MOVING MEDITATION EXERCISE

Moving meditation is a meditative practice done while moving your body, usually in a slow, flowing, repetitive way. It is a great alternative for people with severe anxiety, ADD, and other conditions that prevent them from achieving a calm state of mind while being still.

Before starting, select music or a recording of sounds that inspires you. Ideally, something about ten minutes long. I love Middle Eastern and North African rhythms to meditate in the morning (invigorating) and sounds with traditional South American flutes and wind instruments late at night (calming). Select a quiet space that's free from distractions, whether indoors or out-doors.

- Turn on the music and focus on the sound. Notice the sensations and emotions the music evokes in you.
- As you feel inspired, let your body move in an organic way. Flow with the sounds. Eventually, find a slow move-ment, or a series of movements, that you can repeat for the duration of the music. However, if a specific movement doesn't come naturally, do a basic yoga sun salutation sequence.
- Once you feel like you're in the flow between movement and sound, close your eyes, and repeat the following mantras, either out loud or in your head:

  I am free.
  I am safe.
  I am capable.
  I am strong.

  Feel free to replace these with your own positive phrases if you like.
- With your eyes still closed, visualize healing energy flow-ing through your body. With each mantra, feel another part of your body become flooded with this warm, loving, healing energy.
- When the sound or music comes to an end, slow the movement of your body until you come to a full stop.
- Place your hands on your chest and belly and take a deep breath, thanking yourself for the beautiful practice you experienced today.
- When you're ready, open your eyes and continue with the rest of your day.

VISUALIZATION EXERCISE

This is one of the easiest visualization exercises I know. Ideally, practice this simple exercise for several minutes each day for a minimum of twenty-one days, or as long as you are working on a particular goal. You can easily incorporate this visualization with other spiritual, meditative, and contemplative practices in your arsenal.

- Sit in a calm, quiet place and take a moment or two to check in with yourself and remind yourself how precious you are.
- Take a deep, letting-go breath. As you do, close your eyes.
- Pick a single specific dream or goal you are working on, but only one.
- Bring this goal to mind in vivid detail. Imagine the feelings and sensations that achieving this thing or having this experience will create.
- Without judgment, in a factual manner, see yourself attaining this thing or goal. Imagine it as if you were watching a film or video.
- As you do, again focus on all five sensations. What do you smell, taste, touch, hear, and see? Experience the "movie" of this event in your mind as if it is happening and you are part of it.
- Notice if anyone else is with you in this experience. Who are they, and what do you say to each other?
- As you visualize what you want becoming reality, what positive emotions do you feel? Focus only on positive emotions, and stay with them for several breaths. When you feel ready, end the "film" in your mind, lovingly let it go, and open your eyes. Enjoy!

SELF-HYPNOSIS EXERCISE

While hypnosis is often a guided process done with someone else, you can also practice self-hypnosis on your own. As Grace Smith says, "Self-hypnosis is one of the most powerful ways to reprogram your subconscious mind, and that is entirely free and can be done any time, any place." Grace was kind enough to share the beginning self-hypnosis exercise below, and she offers more free resources on YouTube as well as an app with hypnosis audios on her website, GetGrace.com. As with all these practices, repeat this exercise over and over, and you will steadily feel better with each pass.

- Start by noticing your stress level, and rate it from zero to ten, with ten being the most stressed you can be.
- Take four deep breaths.
- Count down from ten to one, and after each number, say to yourself, either out loud or in your mind: "I'm going deeper and deeper."
- Then, repeat the hypno-affirmation ten times slowly: "I am safe, I am calm, I choose to be here."
- With your eyes closed, imagine, see, and feel yourself being happy and calm for the rest of your day.
- Then open your eyes, smile, and say, "Yes!"
- Notice your stress level again, rating it on the scale from zero to ten.
- Congratulate yourself for improving your state so quickly!

As I say, explore a variety of practices until you find the ones that work best for you. Remember, meditation, visualization, and hypnosis are deeply personal practices, so even as you get advice from others, trust your instincts and intuition to create a meditative and contemplative practice that brings you peace and joy.

4

Yoga and Other Forms
of Movement

Yoga is one of my favorite wellness practices and one of the very first ones I embraced many years ago as a graduate student in New York City. I still remember my very first yoga class: I walked in, asked the teacher if I could use one of the mats the school offered because I didn't have one, and she knew immediately I was new to the practice. I told her I wanted to use yoga as a form of exercise, and she said in a sweet, calm voice with a smile on her face: "Yoga will be so much more than that, you'll see."

At first, I felt like a fish out of water. Most people in the class obviously knew one another. They greeted each other and talked about their lives and the poses using words I'd never heard before, like *asanas* and *mantra*. They all stretched far and wide like experienced and super-flexible dancers. While I tried smiling and making eye contact, no one really engaged with me, so I just kept to myself, observing and taking in the energy of the room.

That's when I noticed that I was unique. Not because I was

new to yoga, but because I was the only person of color. Everyone else looked like they belonged to the same family: slim, long-limbed, and white. I started to wonder if I belonged in the class, but I had already paid for it, I was eager to learn new things, and I didn't want to waste my money, so I decided I was going to go through with it. Boy, am I glad I did. That class was incredible for my body and my mind. It allowed me to tap into a part of me I hadn't tapped before. I truly loved it.

After that first class, I asked the teacher if I could ask her some questions. I was specifically concerned about the chanting and mantras, which sounded like a religious practice, and about the fact that I was the only person of color in the room. In the moment I wondered if I was welcome in that space. We met for coffee, and she reassured me that I was welcome. She encouraged me to learn a bit more about the roots, the history, and the styles of yoga as a way to help answer my concerns. So, as a curious young woman, I devoured information about yoga, and what I learned helped me fall in love with a practice I still embrace twenty years later. I hope this chapter will help answer some of your questions about this incredible practice and ignite a similar fire in you.

A Brief History of Yoga

Yoga is considered both a physical and a spiritual practice, and its main purpose is to help the individual achieve harmony between mind and body. The word *yoga* comes from the Sanskrit root word *yuj*, which means unite. It is believed to have developed in northern India five thousand years ago. It is first mentioned in Hindu scriptures in a collection of rituals, mantras, and songs.

By the time of the common era, yoga was mentioned in religious writings of at least three different religions, Buddhism, Jainism, and Hinduism. A few centuries later, during what is known as the "classic yoga" period, yoga masters from India created a system that included movement and specific poses as a vehicle for meditation and to rejuvenate the body and increase quality of life. In time, yoga traveled to the West, attracting more and more attention and followers.

By the middle of the twentieth century, India's nationalist movement and the fight for independence from colonial England was in full force, and yoga became one way for the country to establish its cultural identity. Afterward, the practice evolved into the many varieties available today, and it has become so incredibly popular and well-renowned that the United Nations has designated June 21 as International Day of Yoga, a day celebrated in every corner of the world.

In addition, thousands of studies have been conducted on yoga seeking to understand its benefits for body and mind. As for myself, after doing yoga for about three months, I didn't need professional confirmation of its efficacy as both therapy and a physical workout regime. I noticed my recurring upper back pain and shoulder knots had eased, and I was able to manage conflicts with less sassiness than before.

However, according to research at John Hopkins University, the benefits of yoga include the following:

1. Improving strength, balance, and flexibility
2. Relieving back pain
3. Easing arthritis symptoms
4. Benefiting heart health
5. Promoting relaxation and improving sleep
6. Increasing energy and brightening moods
7. Helping manage stress
8. Improving connection to community
9. Promoting better self-care

Reclaiming Yoga: Decolonizing the Mind

Those who are new to yoga, particularly people of color, can have lots of misconceptions about what yoga is and who it's for. Those were my confusions when I first started. Yoga was created as part of a religious practice, and for Buddhists and others, it is still used that way. However, yoga today, particularly in the West, is a mostly secular practice. It doesn't adhere to any religion, dogmas, or spiritual beliefs. Doing yoga doesn't require joining or belonging to a particular faith, community, culture, or ethnicity. Yoga is simply a tool to harmonize and balance your mind, your body, your breath, and your inner self.

I had a chance to chat with Melissa Shah, a yoga instructor of Indian descent, who is originally from Brooklyn but now lives in Memphis. Melissa said that, for her, yoga is the practice of being present: "It's practicing this ability to direct your mind from something deeper within yourself. It's tapping into something deeper within you that's unchanging and being able to see and observe things from that place."

In other words, yoga is a very personal practice, with many of the same benefits as meditation. In addition, yoga has many different styles, and every class is different. Some are more contemplative, and some are more physical. It's important to find the style of yoga that works for you, since the rule that one size does not fit all certainly applies here. I suggest researching the most popular styles of yoga online and trying several different classes to see which one appeals to you and works best for your lifestyle.

For people of color in the West, there is the further issue that yoga can seem like something for only elites to enjoy. Melissa said: "In a world where so many countries have been colonized and Westernized, it can feel that way. It makes me wonder how far do we need to trace back to see what these practices really were without the influence of white people?"

We both agreed that we don't have the answer to that question. Growing up, Melissa struggled for years to fully embrace her heritage and culture while living in white American society. "Looking back," Melissa said, "I never actually felt like I belonged, and I also hid the fact that I did yoga after school two or three times a week with my sister, at our family friend's house, or that I was studying to be a teacher when I was in high school and college. I remember I had frames of one of the enlightened beings, and he's kind of sitting like the Buddha, in a cross-legged position, eyes closed, meditating, not wearing any clothes. That was a very customary thing to have in your house, of this being. I remember my friends coming over for some birthday party or whatever, and I hid all of those things. I put them in a piano bench. I thought, they're just going to make fun of it, like why is there a naked man on the wall?"

Melissa said it took years before she felt confident enough to handle those situations and proudly display her Indian heritage. Melissa also now sees her nieces and nephews growing up as second-generation American children with parents who are helping them bridge the two worlds in a proud manner.

Melissa said that she and other yoga instructors of color are embracing the concept of "decolonizing my mind." Like yoga itself, this is also a very personal experience and different for everyone. She said, "If I want to decolonize these spaces, it has to start with me doing that for my own patterning and my own brain. If I'm doing that, then that is going to be what I'm going to put out there as well. I think one way I do that is by always sharing that there's always going to be something to learn, but I think a part of decolonization and helping people to reclaim these practices is forgetting about being perfect at it. Because that's very much a Western mentality that most of the world has adopted. It's not just unique to America. The idea of 'If I don't do it perfectly, then

I don't belong here at all.' If that's the model we're going with, then BIPOC can never reclaim these practices. Because if we're trying to strive to be how the white dominant culture is, how whiteness has done it, we're never going to get there."

I also believe that people of color should feel like they belong, whether in a yoga studio or in a wellness conference. No one has to be perfect; everyone just has to believe in themselves and their own wellness. Since that fateful day in a New York yoga studio, I have practiced with dozens of amazing yoga teachers in New York, Los Angeles, and beyond. I have taken classes in five different continents and have practiced alone in hotel rooms. Yoga comes with me wherever I go because it is an important part of my wellness routine. This is the way those initial yogis wanted it: Yoga is a tool for wellness that everyone can embrace and make their own.

Reclaiming Other Movement Practices

While yoga is the most popular, well-known, and widespread movement practice, it is not the only one. Here are four ancestral practices from other cultures that are being embraced by more and more twenty-first-century folks. I hope you get as excited about them as I am and try them all. They are listed here from least to most physical.

Tapping

OK, let's be real. Tapping is not a workout practice, but it is a physical practice, since it involves tapping your fingers against certain body parts. Tapping is an incredibly simple yet powerful practice that definitely deserves to be reclaimed.

Tapping has been practiced in Eastern medicine for over five thousand years. Just like in acupuncture or acupressure, tapping stimulates the body's meridian points, as identified in traditional Chinese medicine, to help the energy flow and eventually restore balance and health. In the case of tapping, you use the tips of your fingers to tap specific meridian points to get relief from pain, phobias, emotional issues, and even disorders and addictions.

The basic premise behind tapping is that unresolved emotional issues manifest themselves in physical ailments, so tapping aims to address the emotional roots of the problems first. During a tapping exercise, you tap five to seven times on a certain number of these meridian points using your fingertips while concentrating on your negative emotion and reciting affirmations to release the emotion and restore balance. See "Movement Exercise: Reclaiming Tapping" (pages 63–66) for a specific example of this practice.

Qigong

Qigong (sometimes written as chi gong) is a mind-body-spirit practice that uses breathing techniques, movement, sound, and even self-massage. It is believed to help open the flow of energy in the meridians used by acupuncture and traditional Chinese medicine. The student uses slow and gentle movements to warm the body, promote circulation, and bring oxygenated blood to all parts of the body. These movements also help reduce stress and balance emotions.

There are quite a number of qigong styles and practices, and my best advice is to find a skilled local teacher to help ensure your first experiences are enjoyable ones. Qigong is often confused or grouped together with tai chi, which is a related but different mind-body practice.

Tai Chi

Tai chi is one of the major branches of traditional Chinese martial arts. Also known as shadowboxing, its principles are based on the Chinese philosophy of Taoism, which promotes balance between all things and living according to nature's patterns. This dualistic philosophy also believes that everything has two opposing, complementary sides, which is embodied in the yin-yang symbol. Tai chi is essentially a series of exercises that help balance yin and yang, creating balance in one's life.

In the last twenty-five years or so, tai chi has become increasingly popular in community centers, senior living facilities, and even hospitals, especially among the baby boomer generation. It's known for its ability to reduce stress and improve stretching and mobility using low-impact movements. It is so gentle, in fact, that it is considered safe for people recovering from surgery and pregnant women.

During the practice, a series of gentle movements and postures flows one into the next without pause, allowing the body to be in constant motion. Many people see it as a type of moving meditation connecting mind and body, as it is often practiced in silence or with soothing music. Even those observing can feel the serenity involved in the practice.

Capoeira

This amazing Afro-Brazilian dance and marital arts form was created in the 1500s by enslaved people brought to what is today Brazil. In order to disguise the fighting techniques from their enslavers, the enslaved people created dance moves to practice in public, and then they focused on the martial arts components in private.

After Brazil abolished slavery in the 1880s, the government

feared that former slaves would join forces and use capoeira to re-
volt, so the practice was banned. Once again, the people disguised
capoeira as folk dance moves to keep the tradition alive. To this
day, music and rhythmic instruments are an important element of
this highly athletic practice.

. In the early twentieth century, capoeira was taught in special-
ized schools in Brazil, and by the 1970s, it expanded throughout
the world while becoming a powerful exporter of Afro-Brazilian
culture. Today, capoeira is performed by rock stars on stage
(thank you, Ricky Martin) and by young fitness buffs from Miami
to Venice Beach, California.

Capoeira is incredibly acrobatic. It requires dexterity and
includes complex maneuvers like using your hands to balance
and inverted kicks. Capoeira develops a great deal of strength,
flexibility, fitness, stamina, balance, and speed, but it is an intense
athletic practice that requires time to master. It is one of the funnest workout classes I've ever taken. If your fitness level allows it,
give it a go; you won't regret it.

Movement Is Essential to Wellness

Everyone knows movement is important. It's one of the simplest
things in the world, right? We start moving even before we're
born and don't stop until we take our last breath. Yet we often
take mobility for granted, that is, until one day we or someone we
love lose our mobility. That realization came to me when I was
nineteen years old and my maternal grandfather, Papi Jaime, was
diagnosed with a form of multiple sclerosis (MS).

At first, we thought he was just being forgetful and naturally
slower and stiffer with age. Yet MS affected him quickly, damag-
ing his central nervous system and disrupting his body's commu-
nication with the brain, eventually robbing him of his ability to

remember or to walk, talk, eat, and breathe on his own. He died at seventy-five after being bedridden with little to no mobility for almost six months.

The loss of my grandfather was devastating, but I found blessings through the loss. Even as a teenager, I felt that Papi Jaime was too young to die. He was a musician, a music teacher, with a beautiful singing voice and a wonderfully sweet disposition. He was brilliant, loved books, and enjoyed telling me, my sisters, and my cousins all sorts of stories to entertain us. He sat with us to watch cartoons (the coyote and roadrunner made him laugh out loud, with tears rolling down his smiling face); he serenaded my grandmother on Mother's Day with a full ensemble; and he brought Puerto Rican pastries into the house as a treat that we all devoured in a single sitting. Near the end of his life, he was so ill, he could barely remember us or hold his own spoon. The saddest part of this journey was that I felt like I still had a lot to learn from Papi Jaime; I wasn't ready for him to leave us.

That was my first wake-up call, or what I now call a "wellness jolt." I remember wondering whether MS could be inherited. Was I destined like Papi Jaime to struggle with a disease I would have no control over? I assumed that a sedentary lifestyle was partly responsible, and I made the choice then to be more active and learn more about movement.

Our premodern ancestors moved a lot more than we do today. Humans have gone from a lifestyle with a wide variety of foods and abundant daily movement to one with limited nutrients, calorie-dense foods, and a dramatic reduction in physical movement. However, we are still, evolutionarily speaking, the same species, and our bones and soft tissues atrophy without movement.

However, getting a healthy amount of movement does not

require aggressive workouts or spending hours on end at the gym developing six-pack abs. To me, movement is much more about overall well-being, which includes body, mind, and emotions. Of course, we want to be fit, and we want to look great (vanity, right?), but healthy movement is about liberation, confidence, and freedom of body, mind, and soul.

A plethora of research shows how important movement is for our health and well-being. Plenty of research also shows us how bad sitting and being sedentary are for our health. About two hundred years ago, people sat for about five hours a day. Today, we sit for thirteen to fifteen hours a day. All this idleness for hours on end increases our risk for chronic and life-threatening diseases like diabetes, heart disease, and cancer. Every system in the body, from circulation to elimination, is affected by lack of movement and long hours of sitting.

According to the World Health Organization, here are some of the dangers of a sedentary lifestyle:

- Increased weight and metabolic syndrome
- Weakening of muscle and reduced balance
- Increased anxiety and depression
- Increased chances of cancer
- Increased chances of heart attack and stroke
- Increased insulin resistance and diabetes
- Potential for deep vein thrombosis
- Stiffer joints, especially neck, shoulders, hips, and back

Reducing a sedentary lifestyle takes time and discipline, and it involves more than going to a yoga class or the gym once a week. The following tips are meant as a starting point to get moving in the right direction, pun intended:

Movement at Home

- Spend the first three minutes each day stretching a little, either in bed or just next to it.
- If you have a pet or young child, spend time being physical with them before getting ready for the day.
- Get a treadmill, stationary bike, or stand-alone pedals to move your legs while watching TV.
- Walk while doing daily tasks like brushing teeth or checking social media.
- Pick a corner of the house to tidy up or clean and do it while standing up.
- Use smaller drinking glasses or containers to force you to get up and get more fluids.
- Grow plants inside, on a patio, or in a yard and tend them each day.

Movement while Out and About

- Stand on public transportation, then get off one stop sooner than your destination and walk the rest of the way.
- Park as far from the entrance to a shop or building as is feasible.
- Skip the elevators and use the stairs.
- Consider getting a bike to commute to work or run short errands.
- Always wear comfy shoes outside to encourage walking.

Movement at Work

- Organize walking meetings instead of sitting ones.
- Put your trash bin far away from your desk or station and put something in the trash several times a day.
- Take a walk during lunch breaks.

- Get a standing desk.
- Walk over to talk to colleagues in person instead of messaging or emailing.
- Set a reminder or alarm to stand up and walk a little every thirty minutes.

MOVEMENT EXERCISE: RECLAIMING TAPPING

Since tapping is less well-known, I've focused this chapter's exercise on that practice. This is a basic tapping sequence (which I've divided into four steps) for addressing anxiety and worry, but it can be used for other issues. With tapping, the first thing to do is to think about the specific issues you want to work on and their root causes. In this case, ask yourself why you feel anxiety, or what causes it. When and where does the problem come from and where does it manifest in your body?

Step 1: Identify the Issue

While thinking about anxiety, you may come up with many reasons for it as well as related issues. For each tapping session, focus on only one problem at a time. Take a few deep breaths and consider the intensity level of your anxiety. Rate it from zero to ten, with zero being no anxiety at all and ten being the highest level of anxiety.

Step 2: Write a Positive Statement

Next, write down several statements that acknowledge the problem and lovingly accept yourself as someone ready, willing, and able to address it. Depending on your situation, you could write one statement or two or three. Each statement is structured the same: The first part names the problem, and the second part is an expression of acceptance. The exact wording can vary.

The template for the statement is this: "Even though I have [name the specific problem], I lovingly and completely accept myself."

Let's say someone's biggest concern is anxiety related to being unemployed and not having enough money to pay the bills. Their statements might read like the following:

"Even though I have anxiety about being unemployed, I lovingly and completely accept myself."

"Even though I have anxiety about money, I deeply and completely accept myself."

"Even though I feel anxious about not having a job, I am ready to let this go."

"Even though I'm feeling anxiety about my financial situation, I'm ready to face what's holding me back."

"Even though I worry about when my next job will come, I am ready to allow money to come to me."

"Even though I feel anxious about not having enough money, I am open to all the ways this can happen for me."

"Even though I feel anxious about my job interview, I am open to letting go of any doubt."

Notice that the sentences are written with an active, positive tone. They are also realistic and clear. These are essential attributes when it comes to shifting energy and removing emotional blocks.

Step 3: Identify the Nine Tapping Points

Next, identify the nine spots on the body you will actually tap, which are illustrated in the diagram. These spots are the same each time, and they should be tapped in the same sequence as you recite the statements you just created.

Here's the list of the nine points in the correct sequence:

1. karate chop (KC)
2. eyebrow (EB)
3. side of the eye (SE)

4. under the eye (UE)
5. under the nose (UN)
6. chin point (CH)
7. top of the collarbone (CB)
8. below the armpit (BA)
9. top of the head (TH)

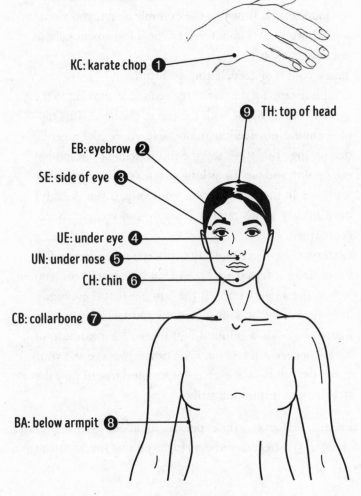

KC: karate chop ❶

❾ TH: top of head

EB: eyebrow ❷

SE: side of eye ❸

UE: under eye ❹

UN: under nose ❺

CH: chin ❻

CB: collarbone ❼

BA: below armpit ❽

Tapping Points

Step 4: The Tapping Sequence

Now you can begin to tap! A single tapping sequence goes like this:

- Using two to four fingers on one hand, depending on how gently or firmly you want the tapping to be, tap the karate chop point on the other hand. As you tap, speak only the first part of your statement — identifying the problem — out loud several times. In the example above, you would say, "I have anxiety about money," or "I feel anxious about not having a job."
- Take a couple of deep, letting-go breaths.
- Continue tapping the rest of the sequence, moving to the eyebrows and ending with the top of the head. This tapping should not feel uncomfortable, more like a gentle drumming. This time, say the full statement out loud at each point, and tap for as long as it takes to complete the sentence. In the example, you would say, "Even though I have anxiety about money, I deeply and completely accept myself."
- Once you have repeated the nine-point sequence five times, take a few deep breaths and evaluate how you feel on the anxiety scale. If the number is still over four, keep repeating the sequence until you feel only at two. Many people do a minimum of five and a maximum of ten sequences in a session. Each time, always repeat your statement out loud at each point, and feel free to vary the statement as inspiration strikes.

Practice this several times per day for about twenty-one days or as long as you need to. Always focus on one specific issue at a time.

5

A Plant-Based Diet

This book is all about helping you reclaim your natural state of wellness, and what you feed your body is paramount to this goal. To this end and supported by science, the healthiest diet is a plant-based diet.

As Dr. T. Colin Campbell wrote in his book *Whole: Rethinking the Science of Nutrition*: "At this point, any scientist, doctor, journalist, or policy maker who denies or minimizes the importance of a whole food, plant-based diet for individual and societal well-being simply isn't looking clearly at the facts. There's just too much good evidence to ignore anymore."

This chapter presents an overview of that evidence, and it provides suggestions for creating a diet that is fully plant-based. That said, I have a personal disdain for proselytizing, and I have no interest in pushing anyone to do what they don't want or are not ready to do.

Instead, my goal is to help you understand and embrace the

healthiest foods for personal wellness and disease prevention, which means reclaiming the simple foods that our ancestors ate and that have helped humans thrive for most of our history. Primarily, these are the easy-to-grow, easy-to-access, and easy-to-prepare, everyday ingredients we are all familiar with: leafy greens, vegetables, fruit, seeds, nuts, and whole grains. Adopting a healthy, more plant-based diet doesn't require unique, expensive ingredients that are impossible to find except in upscale grocery stores (hello, Whole Foods). It doesn't require expert cooking skills, nor do we need high-priced supplements and protein powders, which some people would literally need a second job to afford on a regular basis.

While discussing food and wellness with Jenné Claiborne, a dear friend and colleague who is a vegan chef, wellness advocate, and popular YouTuber, I discovered that the two of us have one thing in common besides a plant-based diet: Both our grandparents ate almost exclusively homemade meals with fresh ingredients and a limited amount of processed foods. Not everyone is blessed to grow up in a family with a healthy approach to food, but no matter what our diet consists of now, we can all learn to adopt a healthier approach. Our life and our longevity, and even the health of the next generation, may depend on it.

As Jenné said to me: "I believe that health is wealth. More than anything else, that's the foundation of any type of success and broader generational wealth. I think it's a requirement. Especially in a country with such expensive healthcare, I don't see how it's possible to be unhealthy and to build wealth in any other form. So, I do think, when you decolonize your diet, you reclaim your health. You start to feel better and to pass down healthy eating to your family and your children. Even for yourself, just having more energy, not having to worry about your health, not having to worry about taking medications — it's just going to free up more bandwidth so that you can do other things and be successful in other ways."

Science-Confirmed Benefits of a Plant-Based Diet

Of course, in this book, I focus on the wisdom of our ancestors when it comes to wellness, but it's also important to take into account the wisdom of modern science. If you are at all skeptical or unsure about the benefits of a plant-based diet, know that recent research supports what our ancestors knew intuitively. Plant-based diets are cost-effective because they are healthier, and they have a positive impact on many of the symptoms and chronic conditions that affect people in the twenty-first century. In no particular order, here is a small sampling of what researchers have found.

A crossover trial, published in February 2021 in the *Journal of the American College of Nutrition*, found that a low-fat vegan diet was more effective for weight loss and had a better outcome for insulin sensitivity, cholesterol levels, and body composition than the Mediterranean diet. For sixteen weeks, researchers studied participants who were overweight, with half of them going on a vegan diet of fruits, vegetables, whole grains, and legumes. The other half followed a Mediterranean diet of vegetables, legumes, fish, low-fat dairy, olive oil, and fruit. Meanwhile, there was no caloric limitation on daily food consumption.

A 2017 review of more than ten studies found that eating a plant-based or vegan diet can help manage type 2 diabetes better than a high-protein diet. Researchers found that those participants who followed a plant-based diet experienced greater improvement in both blood sugar and cholesterol levels, as well as body weight and even mental health, compared to people who did not follow this type of diet. Most of these studies were randomized controlled trials, the gold standard in research.

A 2019 case study published in the *Permanente Journal* showed that plant-based diets are cost-effective, low-risk options that may lower body mass index, blood pressure, and cholesterol levels. The research found that these diets may also reduce the number of medications needed to treat chronic diseases and lower heart-disease mortality rates. The study ends by asking physicians to consider recommending these diets to patients.

The Adventist Health Studies, a series of long-term medical research studies measuring the link between diet, lifestyle, disease, and mortality of Seventh-day Adventists found that their plant-based diet appears to translate to fewer medications and surgeries and less suffering of chronic diseases. This population was half as likely to be on medications like sleeping pills, tranquilizers, antacids, painkillers, and laxatives in comparison with people who eat meat regularly.

Dr. Kim Williams, an African American cardiologist and fellow of the American College of Cardiology, published an essay in *MedPage Today* on his reasons for promoting veganism, based on his interpretation of the medical literature and his own experience lowering his cholesterol levels after eliminating dairy and animal flesh from his diet.

Since 1978, Dr. Dean Ornish has conducted studies on reversing heart disease with a plant-based diet, stress management, and lifestyle changes, with results showing improved cardiac function in just thirty days.

In his clinical research, which is described in his books, Dr. Neal Barnard has shown how a low-fat, plant-based diet can treat and reverse diabetes. This diet has been shown to work better than the American Diabetes Association's own guidelines in treating diabetes.

Plus, other medical doctors, including cardiologists Caldwell Esselstyn and John McDougall, have been researching and actively working with chronically ill patients on reversing conditions and increasing quality of life with a strict low-fat, vegan diet and lifestyle changes for over twenty years.

Plant Protein vs. Animal Protein	
Plant Protein: *Beans, Grains, Seeds, Nuts, Tofu, Seitan, Vegetables*	**Animal Protein:** *Meat, Seafood, Pork, Chicken, Turkey, Milk, Cheese, Eggs*
No cholesterol	High cholesterol
High dietary fiber	Low dietary fiber
Low fat	High saturated fat
Phytochemical rich	Low to no phytochemicals
Mineral rich	Low mineral content
Low calories per weight	High calories per weight
High in antioxidants	Low in antioxidants
Low price point	High price point

Human Physiology: Are We Designed to Be Omnivores?

If a plant-based diet is so good for us, it begs the question: Are humans really meant to be omnivores, creatures who consume both plants and animals for sustenance? That we are is self-evident. But the most accurate answer to whether we should be is: it's complicated.

To varying degrees, human physiology indicates that we evolved primarily as plant eaters. First, we have wonderful flexible hands, naturally short nails, and opposable thumbs. Our dexterous hands allow us to grab large round foods like mangoes and apples, peel a banana, and use tools. Our gorgeous pearly white teeth feature flat molars that allow us to grind and chop plants for easy digestion. Then, the acids and enzymes in our stomach work well at breaking down sugars and other complex carbohydrates and plant protein. Of course, our enzymes can break down animal proteins as well, but those enzymes are not as effective on animal flesh, and our gastric juices often benefit by getting help, such as from other highly acidic ingredients and spices.

Our liver is better equipped to process plants, with a high intolerance for uric acid (a by-product of the digestion of animal flesh). Then, there are our intestines: a fantastic set of organs roughly thirty feet long. This design allows our body to absorb minerals and nutrients, break down debris, and eliminate waste in roughly twelve to eighteen hours, keeping us looking and feeling fabulous.

In contrast, how do we compare to the physiology of natural carnivores, such as dogs, cats, and tigers? Let's examine felines. Their super-cute paws are adorable and not flexible at all. Their claws are curved and sharp, allowing them to break raw flesh into smaller pieces for consumption — which humans need knives to do. They have smaller teeth but bigger, stronger fangs with sharp back molars, perfect for tearing and eating raw flesh. If you've ever played with a domestic cat, you know firsthand that kitty's fangs and claws are designed to pierce flesh (don't blame the kitty if you get scratched).

In terms of digestion, cats possess an enzyme called uricase, which is excellent for breaking down the uric acid produced by consuming animal flesh. Their stomachs also have a high concentration of gastric juices, allowing them to break down the amino acids in animal flesh more efficiently. Finally, cats have very small intestines in proportion to their size, a masterful design that allows them to quickly get rid of the highly acidic waste left behind by animal flesh.

How Much Protein Does Your Body Need?

The USDA recommends an intake of 0.36 grams of protein for every pound of body weight. Under this parameter, a 150-pound woman needs 54 grams of protein per day — the amount in a burger patty plus a small chicken breast. Some experts believe the USDA recommendation is actually too high. So, while experts in the field are telling us to eat less food in general, the average US adult consumes as much as 110 grams of protein a day, twice the recommended amount.

Meanwhile, nearly every plant has some protein (complete or incomplete). Here are some of the easiest, tastiest, most popular sources of protein in the plant world:

- 1 cup of lentils: 18 grams
- 1 cup of tempeh: 30 grams
- 1 cup of chickpeas: 14 grams
- ½ cup of almonds: 16.5 grams
- ½ cup of edamame: 17 grams
- 2 tablespoons of spirulina: 8 grams
- 1 cup of quinoa: 8 grams
- 1 tablespoon of hemp seeds: 5 grams
- 1 tablespoon of chia seeds: 2 grams

If humans were meant to be mostly meat eaters, our bodies would probably be designed more like cats. But the human body is well-designed for eating plants. Not only that, but we thrive on a plant-based diet. All primates are primarily herbivores (most eat insects on occasion), even though our closest primate relatives, chimpanzees and bonobos, are also omnivores. Yet while some primates do eat an occasional animal, they still get most of their nutrients, including protein, from plants.

Animal flesh and its derivatives (milk, eggs, and other by-products like cheese) also have an added disadvantage for us. They promote an acidic environment in the human body, which doesn't happen in the case of natural carnivores like lions, wolves, and domestic cats. Our digestive tract is simply not designed to process animal flesh as effectively, and the length of the intestines can cause the flesh to linger longer than it should, leading to the retention of toxins, protein by-products like ammonia or uric acid (which when retained in large amounts can become toxic), and a highly acidic internal environment.

This acidic environment can then lead to an inflammatory response in our digestive tract and even in other organs. The walls in our large intestine will reabsorb and circulate all those toxins and by-products, leading to a never-ending loop of inflammation. This response manifests in an array of preventable conditions like clogged arteries, high cholesterol, high blood pressure, insulin resistance, metabolic syndrome, weight gain, and early signs of aging, to name a few. These pesky conditions are the root of many of the life-threatening diseases plaguing human communities today.

Hunters and Gatherers: Finding Balance

Exactly when ancestral humans started eating animals is unknown. But starting about 2.6 million years ago, evidence exists that early human species used sharp weapons to slice animal flesh and blunt objects like rocks to break the bones and extract the marrow. Scientists believe that this meat eating caused a significant evolutionary change that led to larger brains and the eventual evolution of the modern human species.

That doesn't mean early humans stopped eating fruits, nuts, and seeds and started eating meat exclusively. Rather, throughout our long history as hunter-gatherers, it is believed that early humans consumed plants and animals at a ratio of two to one. That is, their diet was two-thirds plants, including roots, and one-third animal flesh. This ratio persisted even after humans learned to use fire and developed even more sophisticated tools to hunt and cook. Humans continued to consume a wide variety of foods, and most of what was consumed was from the plant world.

Of course, things changed starting around thirteen to ten thousand years ago, as humans domesticated plants and animals and developed agriculture, which allowed for people to settle in cities and led to modern civilization. The incredible variety of the human diet narrowed as people came to eat mainly domestic crops and livestock. People also became experts in preserving and storing both meats and plants, which reduced the need to hunt or gather wild animals and plants.

For humans in the last few centuries, this has meant that people can eat whatever they want. Or to be more pointed, whatever they can afford to eat. People who don't grow or raise their own food must buy it, and after the industrial revolution, that was the situation for most people in modern society, including our closest ancestors: our grandparents and great-grandparents. This is why, today, the richest countries in the world and the richest people usually eat the most-expensive, richest diets: They consume more meat and more animal by-products (milk, cheese, eggs) than poorer countries and poorer people. However, that doesn't necessarily mean that poorer people are healthier because they rely more on plant foods. In some regions that is the case, but in many impoverished communities, people often have to rely on the cheapest processed foods with the least nutritional value.

Our Ancestors' History with Plant Eating

This super-quick trip through ancient history makes one thing clear: The average person today consumes far fewer plant foods, in variety and in total, than humans have for millennia. In the United States, a USDA survey found that, on average, Americans consume 0.9 cups of fruit and 1.4 cups of vegetables a day, far less than what is necessary to get our daily nutrients and maintain a healthy body. Thus, plant-based eating is not some cutting-edge alternative diet. It's what we need and how we've always eaten.

On her father's side, Jenné Claiborne's family were part of the Hebrew-Israelite community of African descent and raised on a 100 percent plant-based diet. As she said: "Black people, and really people all around the world, have been eating mostly plant-based for a long, long time because raising animals is extremely energy-intensive and not efficient, especially if you can get all of the nutrients you need to thrive from plants. So, people obviously would still eat animal products, but that was not the majority of people around the world's diet, including people in Africa."

Let's take another quick trip around the world to survey some of the regional plants and ingredients of our ancestors. These plant-based foods belong to all of us to reclaim.

China and Southeast Asia

Vegetarian meat alternatives and tofu have been a staple in Chinese cuisine for more than two thousand years, and as many as fifty million people in China are considered vegetarian. Buddhism has had a big impact in Chinese, Japanese, and Southeast Asian cuisine. Eating a wide variety of vegetables is common, and in fact, the population of rural China was the subject of the pivotal "China study," one of the largest nutrition studies ever conducted. In the 1980s, scientists compared diets rich in animal-based foods to diets rich in plant-based foods among people of similar genetic blueprints and looked at the health consequences of both. The book *The China Study* by Dr. T. Colin Campbell and his son, Dr. Thomas M. Campbell, summarized the results, which showed that people with a higher consumption of animal-based foods were more likely to die of "Western" diseases, and the opposite was true of people who consumed plant-based foods.

In countries like Japan, Thailand, Korea, and Cambodia, plant-based foods are also an integral part of traditional cuisines. This is thanks both to the availability of traditional crops and to strict Buddhist precepts, which prohibited the killing of animals and classify meats as a bodily toxin. These countries are also seeing a resurgence of plant-based eating, and their populations are reclaiming their traditional plant-based foods with pride.

India

Plant-based eating is still very common in India. It is rooted both in culture and in the Hindu, Jain, and Buddhist religions. All subscribe to the concept of *ahimsa*, the belief that all living beings have divine energy and to hurt others is to hurt oneself. Kindness and nonviolence toward all living things thus requires not killing and eating animals. In the case of Jainism, specifically, the religion requires a strict vegetarian diet (though they do consume milk and eggs).

According to government surveys, 25 to 35 percent of the Indian population is vegetarian, with smaller and larger numbers varying depending on region and religious following. In the last thirty years of the twentieth century, young Indians moved away from conservative and restrictive religious traditions, and they also moved away from plant-based eating. But today, as the demand for plant-based foods has increased in richer Western countries, so has the desire to reembrace and reclaim the plant-based foods that have been part of India's history and traditions for thousands of years.

Europe

Europe is not well known for its plant-based eating, but that is an unfortunate misconception. Europe's largest ancient civilizations, the Greeks and the Romans, had a long tradition of embracing plant foods both for nourishment and for healing purposes. In fact, before the word *vegetarianism* was coined and popularized, a solely plant-based diet was known as the Pythagorean diet. Pythagoras, the famed Greek philosopher, believed that a vegetarian diet was the best for a healthy mind and body.

The now-famous Roman feasts often depicted in Hollywood films only applied to the richest members of society. The average diet for everyday Romans included a wide variety of plant foods, including legumes (chickpeas, lentils), cereals (wheat, spelt), fruit (pomegranates, cherries, blackberries), vegetables (leafy greens, leeks, beets), mushrooms, olives, spices, and more. The equally famous Roman gladiators were almost exclusively vegan.

A number of Roman emperors and other prominent Romans discouraged the consumption of meat, which was consumed in relatively small amounts. Milk was used to produce cheeses, for cooking, and for medicine or cosmetic purposes. It was rarely drunk in a glass like we do in the modern era.

Africa

African people have been consuming plant-based diets since prehistoric times, and prior to European colonization, vegetarian diets were the cornerstone of the national cuisines in most African countries. The cuisines of Eritrea and Ethiopia, for example, are full of plant-based dishes, thanks in part to the fasting traditions of the Orthodox Christian faith. For Orthodox Christians, abstaining from all animal products up to two hundred days a year is mandatory, so the culture embraced a ton of plant-based dishes. Vegetarian restaurants are common in both countries.

Today, African countries like Senegal and Sierra Leone often top lists of the healthiest diets from around the world. The staple foods and traditional diets of these countries are rich in fruit, vegetables, and whole grains. In West and sub-Saharan Africa, dishes like jollof rice were originally vegetarian (though jollof rice is often made with animal flesh today), and they continue to be very popular, even among the younger generation.

The Americas

Indigenous peoples in North, Central, and South America have been embracing plant foods for thousands of years. South American diets are rich in ancient crops that are now trendy, like quinoa, amaranth, and yucca. The Incas' location high in the Andes Mountains didn't allow them to raise cattle, so they relied mostly on plants and eventually on llamas and alpacas for meat; later, they added fish. The Mayas and Aztecs in Central and North America gave us maize (corn), cacao, chia seeds, and avocado. Both civilizations also had a small group of domesticated animals they used for food, though their diets were primarily plant-based.

Since it arose in the 1930s, the Rastafari movement in Jamaica has believed that food should come only from the land. Called "Ital" food, this refers to food that is organic, unprocessed, free of additives and chemicals, and entirely vegetarian. This Rastafarian diet is followed for both health and spiritual reasons. Rastafarians aim to be as close to nature as possible, respecting all forms of animal and plant life, while the Ital diet is based mainly on the dietary restrictions outlined in Leviticus in the Bible. Ital food is also influenced by Caribbean cuisine, which is rich in tropical fruits, vegetables, and tubers.

Popular Plant-Based Foods from Around the World		
Country or Region	**Food**	**What Is It?**
Caribbean	Plantain fritters	My personal favorites as a child, these are known by various names in different countries, but they are the exact same food. Sliced ripe plantains, a large banana-like fruit, are fried and served as a side dish.
China	Vegetarian spring rolls	A variety of vegetables are wrapped in thin pastry and fried or boiled. Spring rolls are as ubiquitous in China as ice cream carts in New York's Central Park in the summer.
Egypt	Kushari	The national dish of Egypt, kushari is made with macaroni noodles, rice, and lentils, and topped with spicy tomato sauce, garbanzo beans, and fried onion.
Ethiopia	Injera	A fermented, gluten-free grain called teff is cooked into a thin large pancake. Injera is used as the base (and often the spoon) of traditional Ethiopian meals. Topped with beans and various vegetables.
Israel	Sanbusak	This is Israel's version of traditional Indian samosas; the pastries are often stuffed with mashed chickpeas and spices.
Japan	Edamame	Young soy beans in their pods are boiled or steamed and served with a little sea salt. Edamame is arguably the most well-known appetizer in Japanese cuisine.

Mexico	Refried beans	Beans are arguably the most popular ingredient in Mexican cuisine and frequently served as a side dish. Refried beans are usually pinto or black beans cooked with spices and served either partially or completely mashed.
Morocco	Tabbouleh	One of the most popular dishes from the southern Mediterranean, this dish is usually made with parsley, mint, spring onions, tomatoes, bulgur, and lemon juice.
Nepal	Dal bhat	A lentil stew often eaten with rice or other grains, dal bhat is considered the national dish of Nepal and is consumed by the Nepalese at least once per day.
Peru	Quinoa soup	Quinoa was a sacred food of the Incas. It was a seed so nourishing and vital to their health that they called it *chesiya mama*, or "mother grain." Quinoa soup often includes carrots, celery, and potato.
South Africa	Pampoenkoekies	A pumpkin fritter usually served at breakfast, this can be made sweet and savory. Usual toppings include cinnamon, nutmeg, and syrup.
Thailand	Thai curry	This stew-like dish is made with curry paste, coconut milk, potatoes, and other vegetables. It's very versatile and adaptable to almost any palate and often served with rice.

Reclaiming a Plant-Based Diet

As I mention above, my goal with this chapter is to help you improve your diet so that it promotes good health and supports wellness. That means incorporating as many plants, whole grains, and unprocessed foods into your daily diet as possible. Maybe you already do this, but if not, remember: Your past does not define you. If you were raised eating in a way that doesn't support your health now, you can learn to eat in new ways. Your present choices determine the future of your health, your body, and your longevity. So take this opportunity to assess your current diet and identify any changes you feel will improve it. Then make those changes slowly, one day at a time.

While I've painted quite the picture of the "omnivore's dilemma," you may still not be ready to part ways with your favorite flesh-based dish. If so, do not despair. Making changes to any diet is a process that takes time and effort. As the proverb says, Rome wasn't built in a day, and neither will new eating habits be established overnight. If you make changes that are successful for a while, and then one day fall off that proverbial "wagon," so what! Get back up, learn from what happened, adjust as necessary, and keep persevering in your wellness journey, which doesn't end until your last day on this planet. Get back on that wagon, honey, because you have a wonderful life to live and a gorgeous body to enjoy and honor throughout the process.

I know from personal experience, as well as from ten years of wellness and health coaching, that changing eating habits on a long-term basis requires time, passion, a ton of knowledge, and a positive emotional commitment to the process. There is always a pain-and-pleasure dynamic at play: Most people dislike change because they believe the process of changing is difficult or painful (both physically and emotionally). Thus, most change only happens when we recognize that the status quo — staying as we are or maintaining old behaviors — is more painful than the process of changing itself. When that happens, we approach change with hope and the promise of a new, more pleasurable existence. That realization encourages us to seek the knowledge and to find the time and the emotional fortitude to build new, healthier habits.

My experience with veganism has had its ups and downs. I grew up eating and loving meat — things like pork chops, ground beef, and even canned meats. When I decided to stop eating meat over a decade ago, I became a vegetarian for a while (eating eggs and dairy), then a pescatarian (enjoying fish on occasion), and then what I called a "holiday-tarian," or someone who only indulges in meat during vacations and holidays. At one point I even became what I call a "muffin vegetarian." Yes, my diet was 100 percent plant-based, but I ate mostly white pasta, muffins, sugary drinks, and bread. How many nutrients could I have possibly found in that kind of food?! I might as well have been a McDonald's, steak-and-potatoes gal! It took years of education, experimentation, and building better habits that work *for me* to finally commit long-term to veganism.

That has been my journey. Now it's time for you to continue yours. What follows are my tips for changing to a healthier, mostly to fully plant-based diet, which is followed by an even more specific twenty-one-day diet plan.

My most important advice is this: Take any changes one step at a time. This is not an overnight process. Every small step is a step in the right direction. Particularly if your diet has been heavy with meat, don't try to go "cold turkey" or make every change at once. Pick two or three strategies from the list below, try them for a week or two, and see what happens. Then try a few more. After a month or so, as you adjust the balance of your diet and try a variety of foods, your taste buds will evolve. You may notice changes in your mood and well-being. You may realize that you don't want meat anymore, or that meat becomes something you want only occasionally, as a treat or indulgence.

Whatever happens, give yourself time, patience, and self-love.

- Start by eating at least three fully plant-based meals a week. That's just 14 percent of your weekly meals. For instance, pick breakfast on Monday, lunch on Wednesday, and dinner on Friday. Or, make one day entirely plant-based (like the popular Meatless Mondays). If you already do this, then expand by three the number of plant-based meals you normally have each week.

- Make a list of your favorite foods and dishes and see how you can *veganize* them. For example, if pasta is one of your favorite meals, pick vegetarian options like pasta primavera or eggplant parmesan and use plant-based cheeses.

- Eventually, ensure you have at least one plant-based meal every day, and if you already do this, then make it two per day. In my experience, the easiest meal is breakfast. If you drink coffee in the morning, have it with almond, coconut, or rice milk. Or better yet, have a bowl of fruit on an empty stomach, wait one hour, then follow that with a piece of whole-wheat toast and organic jelly. Another alternative is a green smoothie made with spinach, bananas, berries, and almond milk.

- Eat at least one raw ingredient with each meal. For example, if you're eating a bowl of whole-wheat pasta, have a side salad with arugula, cucumber, and avocado. If you're having a Mexican bowl, make sure it includes fresh-made guacamole.

- Use my "reduce and replace" method (for more on this, see "The Basic Method: Reduce and Replace," pages 148–50). Pick a single "junk food" to eliminate or reduce from your diet and replace it with one yummy healthy food you already know and love. For instance, reduce tortilla chips and replace with celery sticks; reduce a bag of Skittles and replace with whole fruit; reduce an afternoon coffee and replace with a cup of herbal tea. Continue doing this each week with other junk food until you have reduced and replaced at least 50 percent of the junk food you currently consume.

- When planning meals, think of animal flesh as a side dish, not a main dish. Make whole grains and colorful vegetables the main stars of each meal. If you still want to eat meat, make sure animal flesh fills less than 25 percent of your plate, so that you are eating less meat.

- Eventually, eat meat only on a single "treat" day. Choose a single day of the week to indulge in meat-based dishes. By doing this, you can also identify how your body reacts to consuming flesh versus whole plant foods.

- Chef Jenné also shared this tip: "Make colorful things, try to show that you can veganize familiar foods, whether they're soul food or any other cuisine. Try to bridge familiarity with foods that you are already used to eating, and clean them up a little. If the recipe calls for a ton of oil or butter, find a way to cut back on those because, of course, it's not just about it being vegan, but it's also about it being healthier. Start where you're at, with what you already know."

- Finally, keep educating yourself. Be curious about food, diet, health, and your own body. Read books on the health benefits of a plant-based diet, and continue to learn the what, why, and how of the foods you eat. The more you know, the easier it is to make the right choices.

About the Accessibility of Healthy Foods

A serious issue that affects most developed countries today is the prevalence of "food deserts" in underserved communities. These are geographic areas where residents have little to no options for securing affordable and healthy foods, especially fresh fruit and vegetables. These food deserts are disproportionately found in high-poverty areas and in Black and Latino communities.

In the United States, it is estimated that 40 million people, or roughly 12 percent of the population, live in low-income/low-access areas with few or no nutritious, healthy food options. There are many contributing factors to this issue, including lack of availability of healthy foods and high instances of fast-food options, transportation challenges (having to travel long distances to buy groceries), and income inequality. Typically, nutrient-rich fresh foods cost more than highly processed fast foods, thanks in part to government subsidies and the food lobby in the USA.

Despite state and local political efforts to solve the problem of food deserts, more needs to be done. In fact, we can all help, at least in small ways. Research the issue where you live, and consider doing some of the following:

- Help fund citywide programs that teach healthy eating and cooking.
- Support bodegas and small convenience stores in their efforts to bring more healthy food choices.
- Support the development of farmers markets in your area.

- Develop incentives for grocery stores to open in underserved communities.
- Support any existing food cooperatives to expand their service areas to adjacent neighborhoods.

Twenty-One-Day Reclaiming Wellness Diet Plan

In addition to the twenty-one-day Reclaiming Wellness plan in chapter 10 (pages 168–82), I've created a twenty-one-day Reclaiming Wellness diet plan. Rather than a prescriptive diet that tells you what and how much to eat each day, this is a collection of tips and advice for helping you incorporate more plants into your life overall. Focus on one strategy a day for twenty-one days, and do it in tandem with the wellness plan in chapter 10. By following these simple guidelines for improving the amount and quality of the plant foods you eat, you will start to reclaim your wellness:

Day 1: Eat the rainbow. There are seven colors in the rainbow. Aim to eat as many of those seven colors as you can each and every day.

Day 2: Favor anti-inflammatory foods. Examples include berries, leafy green veggies, mushrooms, water-based veggies like yellow squash, cucumbers, asparagus, and others.

Day 3: Journal your journey. The best way to learn how the foods you eat affect your body is with journaling. Write down how you feel five minutes, fifty minutes, five hours, and twenty-five hours after a meal to start understanding the effects your food choices have.

Day 4: Listen to your internal conversation. What is your gut and other internal organs telling you? Are you gassy,

indigested, constipated, sad, anxious? How might that relate to what you've eaten?

Day 5: Feed the gut bacteria. Embrace probiotic-rich foods like
kimchi, fermented veggies, raw cacao, and miso soup.

Day 6: Try a fruit or vegetable you've never tried before. Find a
recipe online and give it a go. If you try one each day for a
week, you'll end up with a handful of awesome nutritious
ingredients to add to your wellness arsenal!

Day 7: Power up your breakfast! Add fun ingredients that will
increase the nutrients in your breakfast meals, such as
oatmeal and smoothies. Great examples are nuts and
seeds, powder supplements, and spices like cinnamon
and ginger.

Day 8: Indulge in your lunches. The afternoon is the perfect time
to have a heavier meal or a calorie-rich meal. The day is still
young, your natural digestive fires are awake and working
hard, and you'll have enough time to break down the foods
and utilize them as energy for the rest of the day.

Day 9: Simplify your dinner. Evening is not the time for a huge,
heavy meal that takes eight hours to digest. For dinner,
embrace smaller meals that leave you feeling relatively
empty by the time you are ready for bed. Nighttime is the
time for restoration, recovery, and rest.

Day 10: Embrace healthy sauces! One of the easiest ways to
make eating veggies more fun is to dress them in healthy,
tasty sauces. Some great options include tahini, black garlic sauce, and chimichurri.

Day 11: Drink your water! Yes, water is technically not a nu-
trient, but it is critical to life and good health. Humans
are 70 percent water, so drink it up! And dress it up with
herbs or fruit to infuse it with all the goodness nature has
to offer.

Day 12: Add more alkalizing foods. Because of unhealthy diets and air and water pollution, our bodies have become more acidic, leading to inflammation and potential disease. Alkalizing foods (that is, plants, fruit, seeds, grasses) can help balance your pH and increase the amount of nutrients you consume each day.

Day 13: Choose healthy carbs. Carbohydrates are an important type of macronutrient. Without them, we cannot lead a healthy life. Not all carbs are created equal, however, so the tip for today is to identify which carbs are healthy and indulge in them wholeheartedly. Examples include root vegetables, whole fruit, and whole grains. The rest, you can have as treats once in a while!

Day 14: Plan your treats. Each week, decide what treats you will buy and have available in the house and at work. Some can be naughty, some can be nice. By planning ahead, and being clear about the type and amount of treats you want to allow yourself, you know you will make better choices when the need for a treat arises.

Day 15: Replace sugar-filled drinks with sugarless flavored drinks. Sodas and junky drinks add to your bottom line and your waistline, so infuse water with slices of fruit or herbs like fennel, ginger, or chamomile. Create your own flavorful, nutrient-rich beverages. It's a great win-win!

Day 16: Plan ahead and cook some of your meals for the upcoming week. Once you get into an ongoing routine, it works well to do this on weekends. On Friday: Select your dinners, review the recipes, and make a list of ingredients. On Saturday: Shop for the ingredients and prepare them. On Sunday: Cook the dishes and pack them in individual containers to eat throughout the week.

Day 17: Eat Mother Earth, not human-made. That's right! From

80 to 90 percent of what goes in our beautiful bodies should be natural products straight from the earth, not processed products that cause more long-term harm than good.

Day 18: Practice portion control, and avoid portion distortion. Use smaller plates to serve your meals, and remember that a well-balanced meal with a wide variety of whole foods should provide most of the nutrients you need to thrive. Slowly reducing your portions (start by eating 20 percent less), along with the other tips in this chapter, can help you reduce portion distortion and feel satisfied with every meal.

Day 19: Embrace liquid meals. Liquid meals like green juices, smoothies, stews, and soups are a fantastic way to get a ton of nutrients in easy-to-digest formats. The long cooking process (in the case of stews and soups) and blending (juices and smoothies) act as a sort of predigestion, breaking down the ingredients while still retaining a lot of the nutrients.

Day 20: Slow down to eat. Allow time for saliva to cover each bite. Chew your food longer. This can help increase the number of enzymes traveling from your saliva, which especially helps digest carbohydrates. This also improves your eating experience as you enjoy the flavors in each bite. Slowing down can also help you eat less.

Day 21: Embrace a healthy tracker app like the Daily Dozen (created by NutritionFacts.org). This is one of my favorite apps, as it helps track your daily intake of all the essential nutrients and foods you should be consuming each day. Try this one or find another that works for you!

Plant-Based Activists

Several famous social justice activists throughout history have been vegetarian or vegan. Rosa Parks, Dolores Huerta, Angela Davis, Martin Luther King Jr., and Mahatma Gandhi have been vegetarians. They and others have helped expose the abuses in animal agriculture while simultaneously fighting for human rights and social change.

Veganism could solve world hunger! Multiple studies have shown that if we grew crops for direct human consumption (instead of growing crops to feed animals, and then consuming those animals), we could feed an additional four billion humans.

Plant-based eating is great for the environment! Livestock and their by-products account for 51 percent of all greenhouse gas emissions worldwide, and animal agriculture is responsible for up to 91 percent of the Amazon rain forest destruction (the lungs of the world). Considering this, it is not hard to realize how eating less meat can improve our current environmental issues.

6

Oil, Water, and Heat

As a child of the Caribbean and the tropics, I absolutely love heat and humidity. I may be in the minority on this, but I can't deny it. As you can imagine, once I moved to New York City in my early twenties, I struggled with the weather tremendously. In mid-September, when the New York weather turned cool, I started to feel a bit sad. I mourned the end of the summer heat and the changing of seasons. It always felt like an eternity until May arrived, when I would feel hope again. Those hot and humid summer days in New York City were my happiest ones each and every year.

How much do I love warmth? For years, and I mean *years*, I kept a tiny, secret area heater by my feet in my New York office. I did the same thing when I left the corporate world and started working from home. That little heater has been my constant companion ever since, keeping me warm in the early mornings and late afternoon until the weather is about 79 degrees outside. Yes, I'm a bit of a heat freak and proud of it!

In fact, many popular wellness practices apply some combination of heat, water, and oil to the body to foster healing and well-being, and I have always embraced them wholeheartedly. These practices include saunas, steam rooms, sweat lodges, hot-oil massage, and aromatherapy, to name a few, which can be used to help with pain relief, weight loss, improved circulation, and more. Most of all, they feel good. A hot sauna or massage melts our cares away. Plus, these techniques are easy to use, easy to access, and relatively inexpensive, and I encourage you to explore them all to discover which ones you prefer. Surprise, surprise: I get more excited about those involving dry heat versus wet, but they all work.

The Benefits of Heat, Water, and Oil

Why have people been doing these things for centuries? Here is an overview of some of the main health benefits, which have been confirmed by hundreds of research papers. This list isn't comprehensive, and I encourage you to learn more, particularly if you have a specific symptom or ailment you are trying to address.

Circulation

To me, one of the most important benefits of heat-based therapies is that they improve circulation, which affects every organ and system in our body. By increasing the circulation of oxygenated blood, we can help reduce blood pressure and avoid developing high blood pressure, which can lead to heart disease. On average in the United States, three million people are diagnosed with heart disease each year.

Immune Function

The enhanced detoxification achieved during sweating in saunas and steam rooms is believed to reduce the incidence of the common cold and flu, and it can improve the immune response in otherwise healthy individuals.

Weight Loss

Sweating helps burn calories as the body works to cool itself off during a trip to the sauna or steam room. Heat can also help improve metabolic function, making the body more efficient at burning calories. Of course, for weight loss, this should be combined with regular exercise and a healthy diet.

Detoxification

Sweating is an integral part of the body's natural detoxification process. Skin is the largest elimination organ, and it plays a pivotal role in pushing toxins and pollutants out through sweat. This allows other elimination organs, like the kidneys, liver, and colon, to work better as well. However, this process can stop working efficiently if the body has stored excessive chemicals and pollutants over the years, which is why heat therapies can help.

Inflammation Reduction

Applying some oils to the skin may have an anti-inflammatory effect. This can help in a variety of ways, from calming rashes to providing antioxidant properties to help with many chronic conditions.

Skin Nourishment

Many types of oils, particularly those infused with essential oils and botanicals, are well known to help hydrate, tighten, heal, and improve the appearance and elasticity of the skin. Just like today, our ancestors also used oils for beauty and skin improvements.

Pain Relief

The various combinations of heat, water, and oil have been used for thousands of years to help relieve pain. Steam rooms, saunas, pools, and scented oils can help the muscles stretch, relax, and push out the chemicals and toxins that can lead to pain and inflammation. These therapies can help us recover faster from injury, and they are useful for common conditions like arthritis, musculoskeletal injuries, and some conditions of the nervous system.

Stress Relief and Psychological Benefits

The emotional and mental health benefits of all these therapies are well-known. We can feel amazing after spending time in a sauna or steam room, and scientific research has established why: Sauna use can increase dopamine, a neurotransmitter that improves mood and increases energy and a sense of calm. It also increases endorphins, also known as "happy hormones." Meanwhile, aromatherapy — or using oils infused with various herbs, flowers, and scents — has been shown to help manage and reduce stress and anxiety, especially when combined with other therapies, like massage, steam rooms, and so on. These therapies can also improve sleep; lavender-infused oils, for example, are particularly helpful, whether added to a hot bath or rubbed behind the ears.

Reclaiming Heat- and Water-Based Wellness Practices

Ah, heat! Very few things make me happier than heat. Dry or wet, all heat is fantastic to me. This section surveys many of the ways that heat and water are used as thermal medicine, or the manipulation of temperatures in the body or the environment for cleansing, healing, and the treatment of diseases. Going back to the earliest practices of medicine, almost every culture around the world has used thermal medicine.

One well-known example is natural hot springs, where hot water bubbles up naturally from underground. These exist in every region of the world, and people have always used them to treat a variety of health conditions. In addition to being extremely hot, these waters also have minerals and other ingredients that can help improve skin conditions, relieve arthritis pain, and heal other maladies.

Here is another brief tour of well-known practices from around the world.

Korean Jjimjilbang

The traditional Korean jjimjilbang (pronounced "jim-jill-bang") is a large public bathhouse that originated in South Korea. They include kiln saunas, hot tubs, treatment areas, and showers and have been around since the fifteenth century. Originally, all jjimjilbangs were gender-segregated, with dedicated areas for men and women. This practice continues in most locations today, though some now offer unisex time periods. Further, the bathing and sauna areas typically feature thematic rooms with varying degrees of heat and products like jade, sea salt, and other minerals to induce healing.

Korean spas are now a fixture in most major cities around the world, and they are often run by Koreans with experience in the practice. They retain many original features and practices, such as skin scrubbing, massage, and heated floors and rooms. Modern amenities might include health-food cafeterias, facials, and products for sale. Best of all, many offer twenty-four-hour services and have very affordable entrance fees (which can be as low as twenty-five dollars).

Russian Banya

The earliest mention of Russian banyas — which literally means "bathhouse" in Russian — dates back to 950 CE. The original bathhouses were separate from the main home and often used fire to provide the heat. They had a stove with large stones that then were lifted with a big iron rod and placed in a tub made of wood, creating either a steam or dry-heat "bath." The bather removed the fire and let out the smoke before using the room.

Traditionally, a proper banya involved two main components: First, the person alternated between heating and cooling the body by getting outside in the cold or jumping into ice-cold waters and then warming again in hot steam. Modern banyas use a deep tub or small pool with crazy freezing water. This process was believed to revive the soul — and at the very least, it wakes you the heck up! Second, practitioners lashed users with birch and oak branches to remove impurities and detoxify the body. This is still done today, but typically branches of eucalyptus, linden, and juniper are used. The original banya rooms were used by both men and women together, but after the 1850s, they became gender-segregated.

Laos Sauna Therapy

Laos is a small country in Southeast Asia where saunas are so popular that even the smallest villages feature at least one. They are particularly popular among women, who traditionally used them after childbirth to help aid in the healing and purification process. While facilities are relatively rudimentary by Western standards, the saunas are just as effective.

Laos steam rooms often include a blend of over a dozen medicinal herbs, including lemongrass, eucalyptus, and rosemary, along with hour-long massages. These saunas are places for community gathering and networking and, in many cases, remain a sanctuary for women in Laotian society.

Indian Ayurvedic Sauna

The Ayurveda tradition considers sweating as essential to good health as the food we eat. Ayurveda has specifically perfected the art of using heat in combination with substances like oils and botanicals to help carry nutrients in and out of the body through the skin, our largest elimination organ. Ancient Ayurvedic scripts describe dozens of ways to induce sweating; this helps remove toxic waste from internal organs and protects the skin, which is known in Ayurveda as the third kidney.

An important note regarding Ayurveda and heat is that this practice recognizes both excessive heat and not enough heat within the body as imbalances, and there are protocols to help balance both extremes. In addition, Ayurveda encourages users to heat up the body while keeping the head as cool as possible, to avoid aggravating the "mental home." This is traditionally done by sitting in a "steam box" filled with herbs specific to each person's constitution (or dosha) for about ten to twenty minutes. This is often done soon after an herb-infused oil massage. After each treatment, the user rehydrates and cools off by drinking teas made of rose, mint, or hibiscus.

Turkish Hammams

A Turkish hammam — the word means "spreader of warmth" — is a type of bathhouse and sauna that became very popular in the sixteenth century during the Ottoman Empire, although it's been around much longer all over the Middle East and North Africa. They were originally used as a way to cleanse physical impurities before entering a mosque, and they were often located next door to one. Ancient hammams were designed with impeccable architecture and gorgeous interiors using traditional Middle Eastern mosaic art with inscriptions from the Koran. Examples of highly decorated hammams can be found in Turkey, Morocco, Jordan, Algeria, Lebanon, and other countries.

Hammams were essentially a blend of Roman and Ottoman bathing traditions. Like traditional Korean spas, they were enjoyed by both sexes, but genders were kept separate, and people engaged in other wellness practices, like massage, skin scrubbing, and bathing with the famous black soap — a yummy soap also popular in Africa and made with eucalyptus and olive oils and macerated olives. At the end of each treatment, the visitor could reenergize in a resting lounge with warming tea and sweet treats before heading home. Today, Turkish hammams are not as popular in the West as Korean spas, but I highly recommend them. The experience is just fantastic.

Egyptian Baths

The ancient Egyptians truly had it going on. They were far ahead of their time in almost every respect, and thermal medicine was no exception. Their tradition of using hot and cold waters for therapeutic purposes dates back to 2000 BCE. The Egyptians were obsessed with cleanliness. They bathed in hot water as often as four times a day, and it didn't matter that they lived in one of the hottest corners of the world.

Egyptians believed that clean and well-oiled people were closer to the gods. Their tubs were heated by placing hot rocks in water-filled calderas, and they used soaps made with clay and herbs. While the general population bathed in the Nile River, well-off folks had their own bathrooms! That's right, the ancient Egyptians were the first people to have rooms dedicated exclusively to cleaning and other bodily purposes, thousands of years before the development of modern plumbing.

They were so obsessed with using heat, steam, and water that they had multistory buildings with rooms and whole floors dedicated to different kinds of steam, aromatherapy, and therapeutic ointments and oil applications. Both men and women could exercise or get specific medical treatments. It truly makes me wish I was around during that amazing time in history.

Roman Baths

Probably the most well-known type of communal baths in history, Roman baths were a mainstay of ancient Roman culture and available in every city throughout the empire. Buildings were often enormous complexes with a wide variety of rooms used for bathing, reading, socializing, and relaxing. The largest Roman cities had bigger complexes with fine mosaic decor, marble walls, and statues. The complexes almost always included an open-area pool, dry-heated rooms, steam rooms, cooling and treatment rooms, and an area for working out and changing.

One of the coolest things about Roman baths is that they were available to all — rich and poor, men and women. They had a very low entrance fee on most days and were free during holidays. However, different than most of the other traditional saunas mentioned here, Roman baths were rarely used for treatment and healing purposes. The waters in the complexes were not renewed or drained regularly. Records show the emperor Marcus Aurelius complained of dirt and bacteria, and people risked gangrene if they visited the baths with an open wound. Plus, they were so incredibly popular and crowded that the noise alone prevented users from truly relaxing and enjoying the therapeutic benefits.

Finnish Saunas

Finnish saunas made the 2020 UNESCO Intangible Cultural Heritage List, and they are believed to have been around since 7000 BCE. Traditionally, the walls of the deep wooden baths were lined with naturally bacteria-resistant dust and so clean that women used them as delivery rooms.

In fact, Russian and Finnish sauna practices are very similar. In Finland, people alternate between sweating profusely in the saunas and running outside to rub their skin with balls of snow to wipe off sweat and dead skin, then repeating the process several times. This has a cleansing and detoxifying effect believed to improve health. In addition, Finnish sauna users smack themselves with tree branches for massage and circulatory and skin stimulation.

Today, there is a friendly competition between Russians and Finns regarding who perfected the European style of sauna / steam baths, especially since their purpose and style are nearly identical. Suffice to say, both are amazing, and if you have a chance to try them, maybe you can settle this dispute.

Aztec Sweat Lodges

Living in what is now Mexico and Central America, the Aztecs were the first peoples in the Americas to use heat for cleansing purposes. This advanced civilization was well aware of how important water is to all aspects of wellness, and they created a system of canals that, in my estimation, were even more efficient than the famous Roman aqueducts. These canals supplied residents of major cities with water for daily use, transportation, irrigation, and waste removal, and the waters were filtered regularly. The system was so advanced, private homes had their own baths for individual family use, and women used them before, during, and after childbirth.

Similar to the Egyptians, the Aztecs used a type of sweat lodge, what they called a *temazcal*, along with aromatherapy for ritual and healing purposes. Temazcals were used after physical conflict or battle to aid warriors in the healing process, to heal an illness, and to aid women during childbirth. The Aztecs considered temazcal rituals a way to enable both spiritual and healing experiences. The dome-shaped lodges were typically small and dark, and well-experienced elders guided the ceremonies and placed hot rocks in the center of the room. A little water was then added to the rocks, creating a steam that remained in the well-insulated lodge.

The modern version of the Aztec sweat lodge has become one of the most popular heat-related practices in the modern wellness world today. The combination of extreme heat, a dark environment, music or sound, and aromatherapy causes the body to sweat profusely and purify at a physical level while potentially allowing a mystical and spiritual experience for the user. Many young professionals, particularly from Europe and North America, travel far to seek elder Indigenous shamans who still offer this sweat-lodge experience. Many claim it helps them heal from trauma and clears the way for a more successful, happy life.

Reclaiming Oil-Based Wellness Practices

Ah, oils! There's a special place in my heart for oils. They can be infused, highly concentrated, or simply extracted from my favorite seeds and nuts (sesame and coconut). In any form, oils are a fantastic part of my wellness routine, and they can easily become an inexpensive, highly effective part of yours. They are not only great to help you manage specific symptoms or conditions, but they can be incredible tools to learn about your body and the healing power of touch.

Some like to refer to our skin as our second stomach. That is because our skin is an incredible, porous, stretchable organ that both absorbs and eliminates. We absorb through our skin roughly 20 percent of everything that enters our body. Thus, the skin takes quite a lot of abuse, from the water we use to bathe in to the products we put on. The good, the bad, and the ugly all interact with our skin in one way or another, and it needs to be protected, nourished, and balanced as often as possible. To me, this is one of the most important roles for oils in modern wellness practices.

Oils not only help the skin; they can also help carry the medicinal properties of botanicals into our body. I believe oils are one of the easiest ways to get introduced to the world of wellness, both financially and because of their ease of use. If you don't already, I strongly encourage you to incorporate oils in your wellness routine.

In addition, humans have been using oils externally for healing and wellness since the times of the Egyptians, who were pioneers. They used oils, especially essential oils, in healing modalities and for spiritual relaxation, cosmetics, embalming, and even mummification of the dead. Of all ancient civilizations, the Egyptians perfected the art of using essential oils, and Cleopatra was their biggest, most famous fan.

These ancient Egyptian practices then migrated north through ancient Europe, where other methods of using essential oils were developed. The ancient Greeks believed that aromatic baths and oil massages promoted good health, and they experimented with oils in various therapies and treatments, including surgery. In ancient Rome, gladiators treated their injuries with various types of oils.

Meanwhile, in China, people developed modalities for using oil as medicine and to carry medicine to different parts of the body. Still today, the Chinese consider the oils in a plant as similar to blood in an animal, making it critical and inherent to life. They believe oil from plants can help nourish the blood, activate the flow of energy, and heal the body. They also prepare medicinal blends using herb-infused oils.

In India, Ayurvedic healers perfected the art of massaging oils in different parts of the body for various healing purposes. In fact, it is believed that what we know today as massage therapy had its beginnings in ancient India. Ayurvedic medicine practitioners believe that massaging with oil can restore balance so that the body can heal naturally.

Types of Oils for Wellness

As I've noted, this chapter focuses on the external uses of oil, water, and heat, so this section doesn't describe the many ways oils are used internally to carry medicines and botanical compounds into the body. Here are three basic types of oils that are used externally.

Carrier Oils

Carrier oils are also known as base oils, and they are used to dilute highly concentrated oils or liquids. They are called "carrier" oils because they do exactly that: They carry essential or concentrated oils, making it easy to distribute the additives they carry into the skin. They are also used as a safety precaution, since some concentrated oils can irritate the skin and nasal passages if they come in direct contact with the skin. Cosmetics and beauty products often use carrier oils. Some of the most popular oils include coconut, almond, sesame, olive, and grapeseed, but there are dozens more.

Herbal Oils

Carrier oils are also infused with plants, allowing the chemical compounds of the plant to permeate into the oil. A perfect example of herbal oils is when chefs add fresh thyme, oregano, or rosemary to a bottle of olive oil and let those herbs sit in the oil for several weeks. When ready, the oil will smell and taste a little like those herbs, making dishes yummier.

Essential Oils

Essential oils are created when specific compounds are extracted from plants through one of several complicated and often expensive processes, like distillation, cold pressing, or mechanical extraction. Once those compounds are separated, they are mixed into small amounts of carrier oil and bottled. Some essential oils can be ingested but most cannot.

Methods of Using Oils for Wellness

These various types of oils can be used alone or in combination using a variety of methods, from direct application to inhalation. Here are the most common and easiest methods.

Massage

Massage is one of the most popular wellness practices today, and I could write a whole book on the wide variety of styles and health benefits. Massage therapy can use all three types of oils (carriers, herbal, and essential) in various ways to help the body relax and to promote balance and healing. While massage is often done by an expert, it can also be self-administered. See "Warm-Oil Massage (Abhyanga)" (pages 111–13) for one way to reclaim oil-based massage.

Baths

When you add drops of essential oil or a few teaspoons of herbal oils to your bath, the water helps carry the oils into your skin. You also get the benefit of inhaling the oil's scent. As many already know, this can be incredibly relaxing and rejuvenating.

Compresses

A compress is essentially a piece of cloth or towel soaked in fluid (often water) that has been either heated or cooled. Then the soaked cloth is applied to the skin. The cloth can also be infused with several drops of oil (usually essential or herbal oils) to help convey the oil's healing properties into the skin. Oil-infused compresses can help with a variety of conditions, from bruises and wounds to injury and pain.

Room Diffusion

Diffusion, usually using essential oils, is the most common form of aromatherapy. In most cases, heat and a carrier substance (like oil or water) help carry or diffuse the droplets of essential oil into the room, allowing the user to enjoy the aroma and benefits. There are hundreds of diffusers you can use, including candles, glass jars with herbal oil, and ceramic dispensers that heat the oil using candles or electricity.

Direct Inhalation

Direct inhalation typically involves applying a few drops of essential oil directly onto your hands, rubbing them together, and cupping your hands in front of your face, then taking deep inhalations. After four or five deep breaths, you usually rub the excess oil on the neck, wrists, and upper chest. Note that this is only done with mild oils that will not cause skin irritation.

Facial Steams

Essentially, this is a steam bath for your face! This is done by adding water to a pot and bringing it to a low boil. Remove from heat, add a few drops of essential oil, and get your face close to the pot to inhale the oils, while placing a towel over your head to keep the steam from escaping.

Practices for Reclaiming Heat, Water, and Oil

Embracing and reclaiming practices that use of heat, water, and oil are, in my opinion, some of the easiest, cheapest, and best ways to feel better and get excited about expanding your wellness regime. Mostly, all you need is a little time, though many also involve a small cost.

Heat and Water: Baths and Saunas

Here are four suggestions for combining heat and water; they range from free and easy to expensive and involved.

Easiest of all, commit to having a relaxing hot bath at home once a week. Ideally, schedule this on a weekend when you don't have anything going on after bath time. Use a few drops of your favorite essential oil or simply add your favorite moisturizing liquid soap to the water, then soak while listening to your favorite music or podcast. You can make it fancier — with more products, a face mask, and other beautifying details — or keep it simple: just hot water, a little soap, and you. Remember, reclaiming wellness is about improving well-being. If any process or practice takes too much time or money or causes added stress, that defeats the purpose, so keep it simple.

Next, join a gym with a sauna or steam room. Almost every city has multiple gyms to choose from. Even if you never work out in the actual gym, using the sauna or steam room alone can make a membership worth it. Personally, I use my gym membership almost exclusively for the saunas, which I visit five times a week, whether I get inspired to pick up some weights or not.

1. Right before getting into bed, pour about an ounce of warm (not hot) sesame oil on your hands. If you use coconut or another cooling oil, do not warm the oil.
2. Next add three to four drops of lavender, chamomile, ylang ylang, or peppermint essential oil on your hands.
3. Rub your hands together and then massage your left foot first, paying special attention to the space between the toes, the heels, the Achilles tendon, and any other parts of your feet that feel sore or tight.
4. Repeat on your right foot while thanking both of your feet for carrying you through your day and for the journey they will take you on after a good night's sleep.
5. Rub off any excess oil before getting in bed. The feet should feel nice and moisturized, not sticky or so oily that they may stain the sheets. To avoid this, one recommended option is to put on socks.

This whole process should take no longer than two minutes, and it should feel like a welcoming and relaxing nightly ritual. I do this most nights, but do it in whatever way fits your routine.

Warm-Oil Massage (Abhyanga)

Abhyanga is a type of warm-oil massage developed thousands of years ago in Ayurveda. It uses warm carrier and herbal-infused oils to help balance your physical constitution, release toxins through the skin, reduce tension and pain, and generally moisturize the skin. While it can be done by someone else, it can also be self-administered (what I often call a "self-love" massage), and that's the method described here. Do this daily or weekly, and use whatever oils you prefer.

That said, Ayurveda recommends that people use a specific type of oil for each dosha or constitution, but if you don't practice

Ayurveda or know your constitution, then you may not know what oil Ayurveda would say is best. As a general rule, I recommend using oils like sesame and almond if you run cold or in winter, and using coconut or olive oil if you run hot or in the spring and summer.

The massage can be done in the morning before your shower or in the evening before bed. I often do it once a week on Sunday evenings.

Start by warming the oil in a bain-marie or slow cooker. In essence, in a pot, bring some water to a boil, then remove the pot from the heat and place a heat-tolerant glass jar containing the oil into the hot water for about ten minutes. Important note: *Never warm oil in a microwave.* If there is no easy way to warm the oil before applying it, then apply it at room temperature.

1. Place a large towel on the floor where you will be doing the massage. Place the warm oil close to you (remove it from the pot) and add your favorite essential oil (optional).

2. Take a decent amount of oil in your hand and, using circular motions, massage your scalp, the circumference of your ears, and the top of the neck. Note: You can skip your scalp if you're not going to wash your hair afterward.

3. From there, move down your body, using long strokes to massage the large muscles in your limbs and circular motions to massage the joints.

4. For your torso, use large circular clockwise motions, especially around the middle and lower belly.

5. Once your body is fully covered in oil, leave it on for twenty minutes before getting in the shower to rinse the excess off.

6. Ideally, use a natural liquid soap or shampoo to wash your hair and allow the soapy water to run over your body, taking the excess oil but not removing it completely from the

skin (of course, properly bathe the intimate parts separately).

7. Use a towel that's unique for this purpose to remove any excess oil, but make sure to leave your skin feeling silky and soft. A little oil should still be felt on your skin but not be uncomfortable.

After the massage and shower, wear comfy and roomy clothes. Ideally, do this at least two hours before going to bed to allow the skin to absorb as much oil as possible and not let the oil transfer to your sheets.

7

Music and Community

grew up in a very musical household, so I always think of music
and community together. To me, they are interrelated and mutually supportive, and that is why I have combined them in this
chapter. Yes, they are two different aspects of wellness, and I discuss them separately below. But in practice, I find that one always
leads to and complements the other: All music is a shared experience, and every community seeks to express its own voice, its
own music, if you will. All music is made to be heard and shared,
even if it is made and listened to alone, and no practice is better
at strengthening communal bonds than sharing music together.

Reclaiming Music: The Quintessential Healing Sound

Plain and simple, we love music because the emotions it evokes
are pleasurable. Humans are hardwired to feel pleasure, such as

from food, smells, sex, touch, and sound, in the same way that we are hardwired to feel pain. Once we experience something that stimulates our pleasure receptors, we seek it out, while avoiding that which gives us pain. Music, this seemingly simple combination of sounds, harmony, rhythm, and patterns, can profoundly affect our emotional and mental state, and I would argue it is one of our very first sources of pleasure. Music is with us — soothing us, changing our moods and our emotional state — from the moment we are born, making it the quintessential sound for healing in our lives. Even in utero, fetuses can hear and react to sounds and rhythms. We know this because, after birth, babies can recognize their own mother's voice and even music that was played during pregnancy.

Music embodies and evokes the whole range of emotions. We don't just love happy music. We listen to music to help us release anger, feel energized, reduce frustration, invoke passion, and help us relax. In most circumstances, music helps release chemicals like dopamine, known as the feel-good chemical, while reducing stress hormones like cortisol and adrenaline.

Music has been critical to our evolution as a society and as rational, sentient beings. I don't have to tell you that every culture, throughout the ages, has developed its own form of music that comes to define that culture and that helps bring the community together. The styles and genres we are exposed to growing up become part of our identity, as familiar as our own name. Yet music is so universal that we can learn to love and embrace all kinds and styles. Sharing different musical tastes is how we learn about one another, how we bond, and how we expand our sense of self and community.

I grew up in Puerto Rico, and for years, my grandfather, Papi Jaime, was the only music teacher in my hometown. At one point, probably every person who learned how to play guitar in

Canóvanas learned from Papi Jaime. His brother, Mañeco, a sweet, dark chocolate–skinned man with a unique raspy voice — who, as of this writing, is still thriving at ninety-two years old — played the trumpet and loved my deep enthusiasm for music. Another uncle was a wonderful singer. My mom still has one of the most beautiful singing voices I've ever heard, a talent that sadly only gets to be enjoyed by her family and the folks at her church, but that she still expresses every chance she gets. I learned to play guitar, piano, and flute, and I sang in the university choir.

I grew up listening to my grandparents' favorite songs: boleros from the 1940s and 1950s, which was my parents' favorite music. We also listened to quite a lot of traditional tropical rhythms of the Spanish Caribbean: salsa, merengue, and traditional Puerto Rican seasonal music like *bomba y plena*. Not to mention Spanish pop artists like Menudo, Luis Miguel, Mecano, and Fiel a La Vega. In college, I was exposed to and fell in love with two very distinct musical genres: Nueva Trova (also known as "nova trova" or "protest music") and traditional European classical music.

Beginning in the 1960s, Nueva Trova was a sociopolitical and artistic movement that evolved in Latin America to protest the foreign policy and interventionism of the United States, which supported various dictatorships and devastating economic policies. The music spoke of social change, colonialism, injustice, sexism, racism, and patriarchy, and it embodied the plight of marginalized peoples and the hope for a revolution that would lead to a better tomorrow. Even writing these words and thinking about my favorite protest songs, I feel a rush of emotions and a need to continue the hard work of speaking out for silent voices — that's the power of music!

Meanwhile, I was invited to my very first classical music concert in college. This featured symphonic music from the Romantic period (1830–99), when European society was going through a major shift, including the industrial revolution. The concert included pieces by Chopin, Schumann, Liszt, and others. The music was so melodic and gorgeous, I spent half the concert in tears. I loved it so much, in fact, that the following semester I changed majors, stayed in college an extra year, and graduated with two degrees, in music theory and education.

We don't have to be from a culture for that culture's music to move and inspire us. In fact, it's the universal power of music to help us feel that makes it healing. So when using music and sound as a wellness tool, open your heart and mind. Don't just listen with your ears. No matter the style, genre, or sound, if music helps us feel, it can make a positive impact in our life.

Music Therapy: An Ancient, Now Modern, Healing Tool

Music therapy is a field within modern medicine where certified therapists use specific types of music to evoke an emotional response in patients, helping them relax, become open to stimulation, and eventually heal. A growing body of research shows that music therapy can improve medical outcomes and improve quality of life. From pain relief to reducing the side effects of aggressive treatments, such as for cancer, music therapy continues to grow in popularity and availability. This shows how Western treatments and more "traditional" or ancient practices can be combined to support one another for the benefit of all beings.

Music has played an integral role in healing for millennia. Ancient Egyptian scripts — these Egyptians, they had it going on — describe musical incantations to help relax and heal the sick. The Sumerians, the earliest known civilization, painted on their walls signs that resemble musical notes and modulating sound waves. In the Americas, Indigenous peoples used ceremony, dance, prayer, and chanting to heal the sick and to help the dying transition in a peaceful way.

Only in the mid-twentieth century did the idea of using music to elevate mood and help heal patients become mainstream in modern society. By World War II, the United States and other countries were hiring musicians to play at clinics and hospitals where soldiers were recovering. Doctors and advocates started to promote the practice until eventually colleges and universities began offering training for both therapists and musicians. Today, music therapy is a well-organized profession practiced in over forty countries as a standard part of modern medicine.

The sessions are often individualized for the person or group. A therapist may use music improvisation, performance, melody or lyric discussion, songwriting, responsive listening, and other related activities as a way to evaluate, treat, and heal clients.

Sound Healing: Using Vibrations to Foster Wellness

Sound healing is a relatively new term to describe various alternative modalities using sound for spiritual growth and to restore balance and promote healing. Typically, these techniques use sound in a nonmusical way, even when they use common musical instruments. Some examples are meditative mantras and chants, rhythmic drumming, and striking bells and bowls to produce vibrating, wavelike sounds. Yoga instructors, meditation teachers, and other wellness practitioners are increasingly including traditional instruments, chanting, and sound healing in their practices. Though sound healing is different from music therapy, scientific studies have shown the potential benefits of sounds and vibrations produced by bowls and other instruments on our consciousness and mental state.

Sound healing can be done on your own, but in group sessions, a trained practitioner makes the sounds while participants sit still, eyes closed, and allow the sounds to embrace them. Sometimes the practitioner moves around the room and brings the instrument close enough to each person so that they can feel the gentle vibrations or sound waves. However, many meditation and spiritual traditions also use the voice in the same way. Chanting repeated phrases guides the participant into a meditative, peaceful, healing state. Chanting might be the most popular form of sound healing, since it helps the practitioner focus and enjoy a deeper practice or experience.

Popular Instruments Used in Sound Healing

All of the instruments below are original to specific cultures that used them to make music and for spiritual ceremonies and cultural occasions. When used in sound healing, all are believed to help relax the mind and body, reduce stress, and foster a healing, meditative state.

- **Singing bowls:** These have been used in the Far East for over six thousand years. Different size metal or glass bowls are struck, and the different tones and vibrations are believed to foster different states of consciousness, relieve anxiety, and lower blood pressure. Originally, the bowls were believed to connect listeners to the planets in the solar system.
- **Djembe:** This is a West African wooden drum made with rope and leather. Its sound is believed to alter consciousness and induce trances.
- **Gong:** One of the best-known percussion instruments in the world, gongs date back to 4000 BCE and come from Indonesia and China. They are believed to balance the chakras or energy centers in the body.
- **Didgeridoo:** This instrument is believed to be about fifteen hundred years old and was invented by Aboriginal Australians. In meditation, it is used to help unblock stagnant energy.

- **Dulcimer:** Also called a hammered dulcimer, this large string/percussion instrument originated in the Middle East around 900 CE. It produces a beautiful sound that's almost perfect to help calm the mind.

- **Kalimba:** Originating thousands of years ago in today's Zimbabwe, this instrument has a series of metal tines over a wood board that make a distinctive, music box–like sound.

- **Native American flute:** This is probably one of the most common sound healing instruments used in the United States, since the instrument is native to the Americas.

- **Rain stick:** Originating from the Aztecs of current-day Mexico and Central America, rain sticks are percussion instruments that make a relaxing, rain-like shaking sound.

- **Wind chimes:** First documented in China and India but believed to be part of human cultures around the world, wind chimes are sweet-sounding instruments made of various materials and used traditionally to help improve the flow of energy.

Reclaiming Community

Humans crave community. When we are part of a community, we feel like we belong, like our experiences and emotions are relatable. Communities help us feel supported when needed and celebrated when deserved. They become part of our identity, whether they relate to a nationality, a lifestyle, a profession, a hobby, a skill, or a talent. Communities gather to share ideas, give and offer support and encouragement, and simply spend quality time together.

To me, the word *belong* is critical when it comes to community. We want to feel like we belong. Even those who naturally love spending time alone need to feel like they fit in and have the invaluable benefits of being part of something. Community allows us to share ideas, which increases knowledge and insight. It reinforces beliefs and behaviors, which provides motivation. It offers connection, which helps us feel safe and loved and desired. This inspires us to give encouragement and love.

Without community and strong social interactions, we don't live as long or as well. Research has shown that people with stronger social connections live longer, happier lives, while those who feel lonely or isolated struggle with health risks comparable with obesity or smoking. Low social connections are associated with cognitive decline and increased mortality, especially later in life. A study involving over three hundred thousand people found that a lack of strong relations increased premature death from all causes by a whopping 50 percent, an effect similar to smoking fifteen cigarettes a day. By contrast, the stronger our social networks and social relationships, the easier it is for us to respond to stress and keep our mind and body strong.

In a world where people are increasingly isolated, studies show that a healthy social life and strong sense of community are almost as important, if not more, than a healthy diet. According to a study at the University of North Carolina at Chapel Hill, "the size and quality of a person's social ties affect specific health measures, such as abdominal obesity and hypertension, at different points in their lives."

Author Dan Buettner coined the term "Blue Zones" to describe regions where people live not only longer than usual, but also really well. These are places where people seem to enjoy a much higher quality of life than others. People are healthy, active, and flexible well into their eighties and nineties, they smile often, they engage in sexual intimacy longer than most people, and they are generally more content with life.

In his book of the same name, Buettner identified five regions that are the top Blue Zones, and they are spread all over the world:

- Okinawa, Japan
- Icaria, Greece
- Sardinia, Italy
- Loma Linda, California
- Nicoya Peninsula, Costa Rica

How is it that folks from such different cultures and heritages all experience such a high quality of life? Buettner theorizes that these people share nine common characteristics or lifestyle choices:

1. Moderate, regular physical activity
2. Life purpose
3. Stress reduction
4. Moderate caloric intake
5. Plant-based diet
6. Moderate alcohol intake, especially wine
7. Engagement in spirituality or religion
8. Engagement in family life
9. Engagement in social life

Three of the nine lifestyle choices relate to diet, and they are ones we have heard plenty of times before: Eat a healthy plant-based diet, but not too much, and don't drink too much alcohol. Two relate to physical and mental well-being: Move often and reduce stress. The other four relate to community: Have a sense of purpose, be actively engaged in family and society, and embrace spirituality. This formula has been proven in study after study. Social activities help us strengthen our sense of community, and this helps us reclaim our natural state of wellness and then stay well for decades to come.

Ubuntu: A Philosophy of Community

Simply put, ubuntu is a philosophy that emphasizes the importance of community. The word *ubuntu* has its roots in the Nguni Bantu language, which is part of a group of languages from southern Africa, and it literally translates as "humanity." More broadly, it is the belief in a universal bond that connects all of humanity. The term is often translated as a phrase, such as "A person is a person through other persons" or even more beautifully, "I am because we are." Isn't that gorgeous?

I love this term because it helps remind me that I am not disconnected from other humans, and I have come to use this term and philosophy as a tool for healing at a personal and community level.

A similar concept is *namaste*, an ancient Sanskrit word that's often translated as "the divinity in me honors the divinity in you." In the West, yogis and wellness seekers often use this as their go-to greeting and blessing with others. I also use namaste, and I truly mean it in its full significance when I do. My hope is that ubuntu will come to be adopted and used widely in a similar way. I believe it can be a powerful tool for reconciliation and understanding, especially in countries like the United States that struggle with such devastating racial, ethnic, and cultural divides.

Many countries and regions in Africa have their own interpretations of the concept of ubuntu, which is often spelled differently (see "Ubuntu in Other Languages," page 125). However, every term refers to a similar group of values and practices that African people have cultivated for centuries as a way to connect with their authentic selves and build community. Ubuntu encourages equality while also recognizing each individual's uniqueness.

The end of apartheid in South Africa during the 1990s was the first time the philosophy of ubuntu became well-known in the

West. The term was written into the new South African constitution, and President Nelson Mandela and Archbishop Desmond Tutu used the philosophy to advocate for reconciliation, restorative justice, and healing. As the racist policies of apartheid were dismantled, and the Black South African majority population took control of government, ubuntu was promoted as a way to help heal the social, cultural, and political divides with the minority white population. South Africa's new leaders hoped this philosophy could help guide people to navigate and repair the traumatic wounds cause by apartheid. However, asking oppressed people to reconcile with their oppressors was controversial at the time, and it often remains so, but that is the challenge and power of ubuntu.

Ubuntu in Other Languages

Many groups and ethnicities in Africa claim the philosophy of ubuntu as theirs, and they use different names for it. Here's how the term is known in various parts of Africa:

Angola: gimuntu	Nigeria: mutunchi
Botswana: muthu	Rwanda: bantu
Burundi: ubuntu	Tanzania: utu or
Cameroon: bato	obuntu
Congo: bantu	Uganda: obuntu
Kenya: utu or munto	Zambia: umunthu or
Malawi: umunthu	ubuntu
Mozambique: vumuntu	Zimbabwe: ubuntu or
Namibia: omundu	unhu

Discovering Ubuntu: What It Means in Practice

To me, ubuntu embodies the qualities we need in order to embrace, reclaim, and rebuild our sense of community, whether that community is based on race, nationality, religion, gender, or something else. Ubuntu can help us learn, heal, and bond in healthy ways with all people. However, when we apply this philosophy to our personal lives, this is easier said than done. That is what made ubuntu so controversial in South Africa after apartheid: It is truly hard to recognize that we are part of those who have inflicted pain and suffering on us, and that they are part of us. Sometimes, depending on the circumstances, it can seem unbearable or even unthinkable to practice ubuntu in the way it is intended.

I know how hard it can be from personal experience, from when I first learned of this concept. During my very first year as a graduate student at New York University, when I was still new to the United States, I went to a bar lounge with a friend one night. There, I met a young man who struck up a conversation with me. My English was still rather rudimentary, and I didn't know many of the idiomatic expressions and slang. This man was obviously flirting but also drunk, so I was flattered yet guarded. Between the loud music, his mental state, and my thick accent, he had a very hard time understanding me, and in a matter of seconds he turned from flirty to frustrated to almost belligerent. At one point he asked a question, and I responded in Spanish, hoping in vain he could understand me. He immediately started screaming and calling me all sorts of names that I couldn't understand. The American girlfriend I came with immediately recognized that I was being verbally abused, and she responded to him angrily, grabbed me by the arm, and led me outside. As she explained, the man was calling me a "spic," an ethnic slur for Spanish-speaking people.

I was in my early twenties, and being the target of overt racism for the first time in the United States became a turning point. I became very jaded and embarked on a journey of self-study about discrimination and systemic racism in the United States, a journey I'm still very much on. I wanted to understand what caused an otherwise ordinary human to feel both the need and the entitlement to insult a perfect stranger. This type of aggression against people of color is neither new nor uncommon in the United States, but I had never experienced it as directly as this before.

In the aftermath of this painful experience, as I learned more about what it means to be a Black, Latina woman living in the United States, I kept coming across the principles of ubuntu. This philosophy and its principles of kindness, compassion, and empathy, among others, helped me heal my wounds and smile again. They helped me realize that healing my emotional wounds and raising my vibration to a positive state are instrumental for my own health, well-being, and longevity. They reminded me that if I want to be a vessel for education and change, I myself need to practice its principles in my life. I must learn to recognize the inherent good in all people, even in those who don't recognize or honor that in me. Some people may never be ready to embrace the ubuntu philosophy, but that shouldn't stop me, or anyone, from embracing this amazing viewpoint.

In "Reclaiming Ubuntu as a Wellness Practice" (pages 130–32), I list the eight main principles of ubuntu and provide a guide for practicing them in your life. Through active practice, we can support and protect one another, and we can strengthen and maintain a healthy community.

Practices for Reclaiming Sound and Music

Maybe you're thinking, *Jovanka, I already enjoy music and find it healing. Why do I need a special practice?* Most people experience music as joyful and healing, even if they don't think of it that way. All we have to do is listen to our favorite music or dance and sing to our favorite songs. Of course, keep doing that, love! However, here are two practices that focus specifically on sound healing and music therapy.

Sound Healing and Sound Baths

In my experience, there are three simple ways to practice sound healing. Depending on your needs, you may want to try all three to see which one suits you best. What you experience from these practices will also vary depending on your state of mind and intentions. Some people seek only to become deeply relaxed, others find that sound healing sparks creativity, while some have an emotional breakthrough. Note that the terms *sound healing* and *sound bath* are interchangeable. Use both terms if you want to research further or find a practitioner or group class in your area.

Sound Bath Class

Sound baths are usually offered as group classes, either on their own or as part of a yoga or meditation class. During classes, participants often sit or lie down, while the practitioner "bathes" the room in sounds — such as using sound bowls or gongs — for an extended period of time. This allows you to relax and connect inward. Classes are relatively inexpensive and average about twenty dollars.

Solo Sound Healing

Sound healing is available to anyone, regardless of training. When you hum a melody, whistle, or tap your fingers, you are in many ways practicing a type of sound healing. These actions can help you relax, enhance your mood, and generally feel great. You can also play sound healing recordings at home, such as just before bed or immediately after waking up. This can both improve sleep and set you up in a positive way for the day ahead.

Private Sound Healing Session

Most sound healing practitioners (or yoga instructors who also offer sound healing) offer individual and small-group sessions. This is an option if you want to experience this in the privacy of your own home, or if you want to do it with a group of friends. The individual attention is really great, though it is usually more expensive.

Music Therapy: Meditation with a Purpose

Here is an exercise for using music in a deliberate way as a meditative, therapeutic wellness practice.

First, identify a goal or intention, something specific about your life that you want to improve, such as "increase self-awareness" or "improve sleep." Get clear on what you want to accomplish and why, and put this in writing. If after considering it you're not 100 percent sure, that's OK. The practice itself may bring new perspective, or your goals may crystallize with time.

Then, put together a recording of relaxing instrumental music that's between ten and twenty minutes long. You can choose the music yourself or search on YouTube for instrumental videos. When searching online, type phrases related to your goal, like "music to help improve sleep," or type something generic like "chill music." Make sure the video you choose does not have ads enabled; otherwise the video will be interrupted by advertisements.

Once you have music, commit to doing this practice each day at the same time for a week. Choose a peaceful time of day, such as right after waking up or right before bed.

Then practice in a room where you feel comfortable and

safe, and wear comfortable clothing. Once you are settled in your space, either sitting or lying down, play the music, take one deep breath, and as you exhale, close your eyes.

Focus fully on the music. Let the sound waves wash over you. Follow the melody for a while or focus on the rhythm. When your mind wanders — which is natural — take another deep, loving breath and come back to the music with your exhalation. Each time this happens and you return focus to the music, thank yourself, without judgment. When the music finishes, open your eyes and continue with your day.

Reclaiming Ubuntu as a Wellness Practice

The biggest lesson I've learned while exploring the ubuntu philosophy is that this is a day-to-day, hour-to-hour, moment-to-moment practice. First, we accept that there is a bond that connects all of humanity, then we commit to carrying that belief with us and using it to guide our actions as we encounter others and move through our daily life. In my group wellness workshops, I often discuss the ubuntu philosophy, along with specific strategies for reconciliation and emotional healing. I've identified eight main qualities or principles inherent in the philosophy. These are kindness, compassion, generosity, vulnerability, empathy, friendliness, hospitality, and gentleness.

To use ubuntu as a daily practice, answer the questions below for yourself and create a list of possible actions, strategies, and ideas for each quality. This will give you a great starting point and reference for things you can do on a daily basis to practice ubuntu and build your "muscle memory." Incorporate ubuntu into your life, both for your benefit and the benefit of your community.

1. **Kindness:** Where can I practice kindness in my life? Can I say thank you more often to my friends and coworkers?

Can I return the shopping cart to its assigned area at the grocery store or share my cell phone number with an elderly neighbor for their safety? Can I offer a sweet word of encouragement to a struggling stranger?

2. **Compassion:** How can I better understand the struggles of others? Can I sit and listen to a friend's struggles without judgment? Can I offer a hug rather than my own "solutions"? Do I have the capacity to alleviate the suffering of someone I know? How can I extend a helping hand to someone in need? How can I be supportive in a safe way?

3. **Generosity:** Which positive resources can I share with the world around me? Do I have a skill set I can teach others? Do I have time to volunteer and help others in need? Can I partner with others in order to help people out? Do I have material resources I can share? Can I see my relationships as opportunities to give rather than take?

4. **Vulnerability:** How can I express myself to help others understand my story? How can I cope or help others cope in moments when they may feel attacked? How can I share my experience to help others learn and understand? How can I accept criticism as a tool for growth?

5. **Empathy:** How can I understand experiences I haven't been a part of, without judgment? What tools do I need to help me understand the feelings of others? How can I put myself in someone else's shoes each and every day?

6. **Friendliness:** How can I show appreciation in verbal and nonverbal ways and to both people I know and strangers? How can I show up in my relationships consistently and make them a priority?

7. **Hospitality:** How can I develop curiosity about people and things that are unknown to me? How can different people, places, and stories enrich my life? How can my life enrich

others? How do I welcome others into my reality and my life in a safe way?

8. **Gentleness:** How can I slow down and get the whole picture before jumping to conclusions? How can I be softer in my tone, my mannerisms, and my demeanor? How can I communicate with the intention to love?

8

Grounding and Nature

Growing up in a tropical environment, I was very fortunate. The sun shone almost daily, beaches and lush forests were nearby, and I regularly enjoyed the cleansing effects of rain and a warm ocean breeze. OK, I admit it: I was downright spoiled! As a child, I took all these things for granted. Like many people in warm climates, I often complained about the heat and humidity. Then I moved to the concrete, human-made jungle of New York and realized how much I love heat and humidity and how blessed I was to grow up connected to Mother Earth and her many wonders.

My parents and grandparents were not keen on children wandering around barefoot, but they intuitively knew the importance of being in touch with the earth. Growing up, my cousins, sisters, and I spent our summer days at Mami Eva's house. My mom dropped us off before 8 a.m. on her way to work, and after breakfast, Mami Eva announced to the household full of loud children: "Time to head outside and play in the sun." We took our shoes off and ran around, playing and chasing one another in the yard, allowing our toes to enjoy the fresh-cut grass and our skin to be kissed by the tropical morning sun. We were often outside for about two hours before Mami Eva called us back in because it had become too hot to be exposed to the sun.

Those are some of my fondest memories of my carefree childhood and my connection with the land we called home. My elders unknowingly gave me a great foundational gift that many decades later proved instrumental in my healing journey. In order to reclaim my natural state of wellness, I had to learn to get back to nature, to "ground" myself and connect to the earth.

We all have this connection to nature and to the whole world: to earth, to water, to air, and to all living creatures. To me, the easiest analogy for imagining this is mycelium. Mycelium is a network within fungus that's equivalent to the root system in plants. It is like a network within a network of tiny, fine, white, veinlike filaments that provide food and nutrients for mushrooms. Mycelium is both directly and indirectly connected to everything in the forest: both living and dead. Mycelium is responsible for creating high-quality soil in the forest, decomposing dead leaves and other forest debris, providing nutrients to plants and animals, and supporting plant and animal life as a whole. This almost invisible force supports all life on earth.

Like mycelium, we are connected to the cycles of growth, death, and rebirth, and our lives impact, and are impacted by, all other life. Every single choice we make affects not only us but everyone and everything directly connected to us and, ultimately, the earth as a whole. Our ancestors many thousands of years ago understood this inherent interconnection among all life and the need to support Mother Earth's natural regenerative processes. They knew our own survival depended on it.

In other words, this chapter isn't only about how connection to nature improves human wellness, but how humans also need to protect and heal the earth that supports us and all life.

The Benefits of Grounding

Our connection with the earth is undeniable. We rely on Mother Earth for the air we breathe, the water we drink, and the foods that keep us alive and well.

Sadly, however, modern life has made us increasingly disconnected from nature. We spend more hours inside buildings than outside them, and no matter where we are, our faces are glued to an ever-growing number of screens: on our phones, our tablets, and our computers, on our TVs and in theaters. Indeed, many urban dwellers might go weeks or even months without touching any part of the earth. People in urban centers have limited access to grassy areas, sandy beaches, and forests. We don't always have regular contact with natural bodies of water or even get to breathe clean fresh air. Even when in nature, the shoes we wear block direct contact with the ground. Many people don't consume living foods regularly (that is, raw fruits and vegetables), and some have no idea how or where food is grown. Given all this, it's no wonder we're not well! The modern comforts designed to make our lives easier, more efficient, and seemingly happier are contributing to growing incidences of chronic stress, physical and emotional fatigue, anxiety, and other mood disorders. Even when we're with other people, we can feel increasingly isolated and disconnected. I wholeheartedly believe that our disconnection from the natural world is exacerbating these issues.

This is why the wellness practice of grounding, or what's also called "earthing," has become so vital. This involves any activity that helps us reconnect or "ground" to nature and the earth. At its most fundamental, this means literally touching the earth with our hands, feeling nature on our skin. It means walking barefoot in the grass and swimming in the ocean and feeling bark on our palms.

One theory behind the benefits of grounding is that the earth is one giant antioxidant. When we come in contact with nature, our electrical frequencies sort of synchronize with the earth's, which helps our bodies to fight free radicals, inflammation, and disease. Since the 1990s, researchers have been studying the connection between the earth's electrical field and its effects on mood, physiology, and overall health. These studies have mostly focused on issues that affect millions of people — like pain, mood disorders, and inflammation — and so far, most of the data is anecdotal. However, studies are increasingly showing that grounding benefits a variety of health concerns:

- It reduces inflammation, especially the obvious signs of inflammation following injury, like redness, heat, swelling, and loss of function.
- It reduces pain, both its intensity and duration.
- It improves energy in the morning and maintains normal levels throughout the day.
- It improves sleep. Reports document people falling asleep faster and waking up fewer times throughout the night.
- It decreases stress, in part by reducing the stress hormone cortisol, regulating heart rate, and normalizing muscle tension.
- It improves mood, even with limited exposure of grounding for only an hour.
- It increases blood flow. Grounding promotes blood regulation and circulation, positively affecting the look and feel of the skin in the face and extremities.
- It increases metabolic rate, which allows people to utilize the nutrients from food, to metabolize fats and toxins, and to maintain their weight at healthy levels.

- It reduces symptoms of PMS, hot flashes, and other types of menstrual and menopausal discomfort.
- It has anti-aging effects. Grounding repairs free radical damage and oxidative stress, which can aid tissue repair and reduce the appearance of fine lines and sagging skin.

Reclaiming Grounding

Our ancestors walked around with bare feet, slept on the ground, hunted, gathered, and were constantly exposed to water, air, earth, and sun, and from what we know, they regarded all beings, including humans, as interconnected. Most of the world's cultures share similar beliefs. Even just a couple of generations ago, people spent much more time outdoors and in direct contact with nature. In fact, it's so well-documented how much more connected with nature people once were that I will keep this overview brief.

The ancient Chinese developed the concept of qi (pronounced "chee"), which names the life force that connects humans with the earth. Just as qi affects bodies of water, the tide, the weather, and more, so qi affects our bodies, our circulation, and our energy flow. Balancing qi is therefore one of the ways people can resolve physical and emotional imbalances.

Indigenous peoples of Asia, Africa, Europe, and the Americas all communed with and honored the land and all beings. Safeguarding the land and life was an integral part of their spiritual beliefs and ritualistic systems. Nature wasn't something to exploit but was conceptualized as Mother Earth, the spiritual and literal source of all life and sustenance. They understood that nature is both powerful and vulnerable, and they constantly navigated the delicate balance between giving and taking. Most cultures made it a central goal to maintain their balanced, symbiotic relationship with Mother Earth, who both gives and takes life.

We don't need experts and scientific research to confirm that getting back in touch with the earth is a requisite. We know from our own experience how refreshing and important nature is. We feel it after a day at the beach or breathing fresh air during a nature walk. If grounding feels somehow like we're going back to our roots, it's because we are. Reclaiming our physical and emotional connection to the earth is not only important to help us reclaim our state of wellness, but it is critical to help us reconnect with our own humanity and help preserve the world that sustains us.

Humanity's Impact on Nature and Our Own Well-Being

Modern human life has been increasingly and negatively affecting the natural world for more than three hundred years. And we have reached the point where we cannot simply talk about it. We must make daily choices that heal, support, and reconnect us to the natural world. Mother Earth is not well. She is sick and struggling to survive, and since we depend on her for our own well-being, that means we are impacted as well. Today, we know what we need to do. We know how to help heal and reconnect with nature. But we must make the commitment to do so. We must each agree to do our part for the benefit of all sentient beings or else nature will continue declining and making life harder for future generations.

Of course, what I'm referring to is global warming and climate change. While I don't have the room in this book to detail the countless studies showing the devastating effects of human impacts and excessive fossil fuel use on the environment, I would be remiss if I didn't discuss the devastating health consequences that this is having on us, especially in poor communities and developing nations around the world.

The World Health Organization (WHO) has reported that climate change is responsible for the deaths of 150,000 people per year and that number may double in less than a decade. Sadder still, the people most severely impacted by global warming tend to be those living in countries that contribute the least to the problem. So what the richest countries do, those that contribute the most to global warming, impacts the health of our fellow brothers and sisters in every corner of the world. What happens in India and Africa can affect Brazil and Canada. What happens in the United States can impact Colombia and Morocco. That's how interconnected we are.

However, no one is immune to the health effects of climate change. We have only one planet. Here are some of the most common climate change–related threats to our health and well-being:

Infectious Diseases

High temperatures, habitat loss, and deforestation can lead to increased populations of insects like mosquitoes, which carry diseases like malaria, dengue fever, and Legionnaires' disease, a bacterial lung infection. An outbreak of this disease occurred in the United Kingdom in 2006 that scientists attributed to global warming.

Heatstroke

Greenhouse gas emissions — excessive gasses, created by a variety of human activities, that get trapped in the earth's atmosphere, causing the weather to become hotter — increase the likelihood of heat waves, which in turn increase the risk of heatstroke. This condition can be fatal, even in otherwise healthy people, but the very old, the very young, and the health-compromised are especially vulnerable.

Respiratory Diseases

When the weather gets really warm, our heart must work a little harder to keep our body cool. If someone also struggles with respiratory conditions like allergies or asthma, they can be even more at risk for serious health issues. In addition, hot temperatures increase the concentration of ozone in the atmosphere, which can damage lung tissue and lead to serious health risks for people with respiratory conditions.

Stress-Related Disorders

Mental illness is one of the main causes of pain and suffering in the developed world. The extreme effects of climate change can exacerbate stress disorder symptoms for people with existing mental health issues, but it can also affect those without preexisting issues. This is especially true immediately following a natural or human-created disaster.

Pollution

While not a specific health condition, increased pollution due to human impacts is indeed a major health threat to all. Not even the healthiest, richest nations can escape the impacts of polluted air, water, and soil and of overfishing, deforestation, and cattle ranching. As pesticides, chemicals, and toxins become absorbed into nature, they inevitably get into human bloodstreams and can lead to the development of dozens of preventable diseases.

Practices for Reclaiming Grounding

Whether these practices are called grounding, earthing, or simply reconnecting with nature, they accomplish the same thing. Most share an essential element: physically touching or making contact with the natural world. This is an underrated but critical component of wellness: Allowing our body to physically connect with nature fosters emotional connection. We must all fall in love (or fall back in love) with Mother Earth, which will inspire more deliberate efforts to protect her.

Walk Barefoot

This is as simple as it sounds. In a yard or park, it doesn't get easier than taking your shoes off and walking around barefoot for twenty to thirty minutes each day. If you live in a city, find a suitable park or green space nearby. If the area is small, you can sit, take your shoes off, and simply allow your feet to touch the earth without walking. Let your feet get dirty; squish your toes in the mud. If it's warm, wear shorts and a T-shirt and let as much of your naked skin feel the earth, wind, and weather as you can. If it's cold, still go barefoot. Walk in the snow for as long as you can handle without jeopardizing your extremities.

Lie Down

The more skin that gets in touch with the natural world, the better. Get as naked as possible, or as much as you feel comfortable and is legal, and lie down on the grass or on a sandy beach. Warm sand is a fantastic conduit for the electrical charges from the earth. Bury yourself in the sand up to your neck, then clean yourself off by swimming in the ocean.

Submerge in Water

Speaking of water, swimming is another awesome way to connect and ground with nature — whether in the ocean, a lake, or a river. According to experts, submerging in natural bodies of water is just as effective for grounding purposes, though swimming in concrete or plastic, chlorinated pools is not. If you can handle cold water, swim outdoors for as much of the year as you can stand.

Practice Forest Bathing

This wellness technique was originally developed in Japan. Forest bathing involves spending quiet, meditative time in a forest, taking in the atmosphere and surroundings with all your senses. People sit, lie down, touch and interact with the flora, meditate, smell, look, and otherwise use their entire being to become one with the forest. I've tried it, and the effect is similar to those of other forms of grounding.

Garden

Don't have a green thumb? Don't have space where you live for an outdoor garden? Doesn't matter. As somebody with the worst green thumb ever who practiced this while living in a tiny New York City apartment, I can tell you that buying a couple of little pots, some soil, and baby plants and connecting with them for a minute or two a couple of times per day can be highly satisfying. It is one way to reconnect with the earth even in an urban world.

Use Grounding Equipment

Grounding equipment is an indirect way to ground yourself, but in my experience, it is neither as satisfying nor as effective as direct contact with nature. However, it is very popular in some wellness circles, and you might find it useful. It requires buying and using special equipment like grounding mats, sheets, blankets, socks, skin patches, and bands. Manufacturers and sellers swear by their products, which promise to help you recharge in the same way as other grounding activities. Personally, I'd only use these as a last resort if being in nature is difficult in your situation.

Strategies to Protect Mother Earth

The debate surrounding climate change and global warming can be overwhelming and highly politicized, even when the vast majority of scientists and experts agree, based on the data, that humans have a negative impact on climate change. Yet whatever the total cause of global warming, and whatever the ultimate impacts will be, there are still many things we can do right now to lessen the negative impact humans have on the environment.

There is no denying that humans could afford to be kinder to Mother Earth. We might even find joy living a bit simpler and reducing our carbon footprint. With that in mind, here are strategies related to the three things that contribute most to our personal carbon footprint: food, housing, and transportation.

Food

A plant-based diet is the best diet for our personal health and well-being, and it's the best diet for the earth. Growing animals for human consumption is one of the biggest causes of deforestation (the lungs of the planet), global hunger, and water and land pollution. One of the best and easiest ways to reduce your impact on the environment is by eating more plants, ideally in season and from local vendors, like at farmers markets. That way, food doesn't have to travel very far to get to your kitchen. Rich countries are also notorious for food waste: Roughly 40 percent of the food people buy in the United States goes to waste. So, plan your meals to avoid cooking or buying more than you can consume, freeze any unused food to consume later, and share your meals with your neighbors to avoid food waste.

Housing

At home, we can make a big difference by turning off appliances, regulating the heating and cooling systems, and using smaller equipment like laptops versus desktops. If your budget permits, replace older appliances with more energy-efficient ones, and make the whole house more energy efficient with better insulation and roofing. Planting vegetation around a house helps keep it cooler in the summer and warmer in the winter. Finally, participate in your town's recycling program to minimize household waste.

Transportation

Everyone's situation is different, but the goal here is to minimize driving a car. Depending on how far you live from where you work and shop, use public transportation, ride a bike, or arrange a carpool instead of driving a car. Then, when using a car (particularly when shopping), plan trips so you don't waste miles and gas going back and forth. Then service your car and tires regularly, so they are more efficient. If you don't already own a hybrid or electric vehicle, consider one for your next purchase.

9

The Reclaiming Wellness Method

Now that you've learned about the seven wellness practices, you might be thinking: *How do I implement these tips and strategies? My life is already full! I'd like to create a healthier lifestyle, but making all these changes seems overwhelming.*

If that describes you, don't worry. It's natural to feel uncertain and overwhelmed when contemplating life changes. In the next two chapters, I describe the Reclaiming Wellness Method, which is a practical, flexible, easy-to-follow plan for adopting a healthier lifestyle in a way that fits who you are and what you want. The whole goal is to put you in charge. Using this method, you get to decide what you want to do and how fast or slow you want to go. I want you to feel empowered to make the process your own based on your unique lifestyle.

In this chapter, I describe the method itself, which is actually very simple, and I answer the main questions and concerns people often have about whether this method and these practices are right for them. Then I discuss preparation, which is a critical step. We have to "clean house" and assess where we're at, what we want, and what we need first. This allows us to make a practical, appropriate plan that fits our current life, so we can make changes successfully. Finally, this chapter ends with three examples of how you might adopt a few new wellness practices on a daily and weekly basis. Then, chapter 10, "Recipe for Success," pulls it all together and provides a guide for incorporating strategies from all seven wellness practices as part of a full twenty-one-day process.

Go Slow: Ease Your Way In

As you contemplate the lifestyle changes you want to make, the best way to avoid becoming overwhelmed is to go slow. Sometimes, we are so eager to improve our life and feel better that we rush ahead and try to change everything all at once. I can tell you from experience that's not the most successful approach.

After years of struggling with digestive issues and hormonal disruption, I embarked on a journey of healing and self-discovery. My quick-yet-organized vata-pitta (Ayurvedic constitution) brain wanted to learn it all, fast, and I tried to do a million things at once in order to get results just as fast. I tried yoga, visited an Ayurvedic practitioner, had a regular acupuncturist and a traditional Chinese medicine practitioner, completely changed my diet to quasi-vegetarian, took on meditation and self-hypnosis, and went regularly to bathhouses and on trips to the park and the woods. Within a span of about forty-five days I incorporated all of this into my daily and weekly routines. In hindsight, it was unnecessary and a bit ridiculous. I was rushing to heal as if the human body worked as fast as the imagination. That was silly, but it taught me a valuable lesson about the gift of patience and learning to listen to our *body*, our only home, the most incredible instrument we will ever play in this wonderful symphony we call life. This experience was foundational, and it has informed the method I now use with clients, students, and you, dear reader.

I remember a specific instance when, trying to be extra efficient with my new wellness routine, I signed up for a hot yoga class. My goal was to meet two goals at once: getting into a heated room to help me sweat and doing my first yoga class in a few weeks. This might not have been an issue necessarily, except that I was in the middle of transitioning into a super-clean diet prescribed by a naturopathic doctor, and my system was going through a big transition. The class started out well, but about twenty minutes into it, I started to feel faint. I lay down for several minutes and eventually left the class. I was nauseous the rest of the night. Luckily, I felt better the next morning, but the experience taught me a big lesson. My body had not developed problems overnight, and it wasn't going to restore balance and wellness in a week. I learned that it's often better to start slow and with easier practices that help us feel better. This comfortable progress can then empower and inspire us to keep going and improving without burning out.

Listen to Your Body

As you follow this process yourself, listen to the cues your body gives you when deciding what to do. Focus on improving your relationship with your body: both the exterior and the interior, the vital organs you never see. One thing that can help with this is to make any diet changes before incorporating other wellness practices. Remember, you want to be respectful of your body's needs as you transition into making long-term changes.

The process of incorporating new wellness practices into your routine is similar to starting a new diet or a type of cleanse. The concept behind cleansing or detoxing is to replace toxin-filled foods with clean, nourishing foods to optimize the elimination process and eventually beautify the body from the inside out. This process can take a few days, a few weeks, or even longer, but it can initially cause some rather uncomfortable side effects as all that toxicity works its way through and out of your body. Many people starting a new wellness routine or a new diet struggle with this initial period. They feel uncomfortable, blame it on the new routine, and drop it. Of course, once they go back to their old routine, they go back to *feeling like themselves again*, which may or may not be great, but it's enough to believe that the new wellness routine is the cause of their initial discomfort and toss it aside as a failure.

I have heard this story so many times I've lost count. Someone begins a new wellness plan and gets overexcited and overambitious. They start strong, see a little progress — maybe they lose some weight, their skin clears, their stress diminishes — and then ramp up to try to do everything in a couple of days. But they don't account for a period of adjustment, neither in their body nor in their life. They can't keep up with everything they are doing, start to feel overwhelmed, and crash and burn. Many will decide, or friends or family members will tell them, that alternative practices just must not be their thing. They go back to their old lifestyle, feeling disillusioned and unfulfilled, having given up on all the goodness that the world of wellness has to offer. Goodness that is part of our DNA, our history, our ancestry.

So, go slow. Ease into new practices. And listen to your body, which will tell you when it's ready to do more.

The Basic Method: Reduce and Replace

The simplest and most effective way to adopt new lifestyle practices is to use my "reduce and replace" method, which I mention briefly in chapter 5 (see "Reclaiming a Plant-Based Diet," pages

81–85). This is incredibly effective for upgrading eating habits, but it is equally effective for adding any practice to a new wellness routine without overwhelm.

In essence, the idea is that, in order to add something new to our lives, we must eliminate or reduce something else. The key is to focus on taking one small step at a time. For instance, if someone knows they eat too much junk food, they wouldn't try to quit cold turkey and eliminate all junk food at once. Instead, using reduce and replace, they would pick a single junk food to eliminate or reduce and replace it with one yummy, healthy food they already know and love, while keeping the rest of their diet the same. After doing this for a few days or a week, they would reduce and replace one more junk food, and so on, until they had reached their goal. This might be eating 70 or 80 percent less junk food, which will eventually allow them to indulge every now and then without guilt. It will also allow them to get a few added benefits, including retraining their taste buds to newer, healthier foods, being more aware of how their body feels when consuming healthy or junk food, and more.

You can use the same strategy for any wellness practice. Let's say someone wants to develop a daily meditation routine. First, they need to consider their current daily routine and determine when to meditate. Meditation takes time, so they need to identify a period of time that isn't currently being used, or else they need to reduce the amount of time they spend on something else and replace it with meditation. That something else might be an activity that is the equivalent of "junk food," like watching television or scrolling social media. Or it might mean reducing an important activity — say, getting up half an hour earlier in the morning and replacing that sleep time with meditation.

In addition, the person wouldn't necessarily start by meditating every day. They might meditate only once a week for a month, then several times a week, and slowly build to a daily practice over several months. Typically, it takes between twenty-one and twenty-eight days for a new activity to be cemented as a habit. So always give each new activity at least that long, if not longer, to ensure it works for you and becomes ingrained as a habit.

At the same time, we also need to evaluate our life, our personality, and our situation (see "Preparation and Planning," pages 154–60). Adopting certain wellness practices can be harder or easier for a variety of reasons. If we have a lot of stress in our life, this can lead us to feel depleted and unhappy, and it can deter our efforts to make changes and find peace within. However, in the same fashion that we "reduce and replace" in order to add new things, we can focus on reducing the causes of stress by doing things that lessen stress, like meditation or self-hypnosis. Further, sometimes we have concerns and fears about what making certain changes will mean and so we resist change, even if we know we need it. This is what I address next.

FAQ: Is Reclaiming Wellness for Me?

Many of my clients and students come to me with very valid questions and concerns about adopting new wellness practices, so in this section I provide the most frequently asked questions and my usual responses. I hope these address any concerns you may have and help you to embrace reclaiming wellness.

That said, sometimes people ask these questions because they are resisting change in itself. This is natural. Resistance is a normal part of the growing process. Change often inspires resistance because we have been trained to believe that change is hard, maybe even painful. So if you feel resistance in yourself at any point, please do not be too hard on yourself. Most of my students and clients feel that emotional pushback at the start of their wellness journeys. It might mean that you need to proceed more slowly or gently, by either focusing on smaller goals or adjusting in ways that lessen resistance.

How much time will this take? I am already busy and overwhelmed.

Everyone is busy all the time, but I assure you, if you make time for wellness, you will be so happy you did. You will become more grounded, healthier, and balanced, which will lead to a happier family life, work life, and emotional life. Wellness will help you feel less busy, even if you work just as much. That said, pace yourself. If you are very busy with immovable obligations, find small moments and ways to incorporate a few practices. Then expand as you have more time. The important thing is to get started and then go slowly but steadily.

What if I don't know anything about these wellness practices? Can I still do this?

The Reclaiming Wellness Method is designed for anyone who is interested in becoming a healthier, happier, more well-rounded individual. All you need is the desire to nurture your body and mind, and you can learn everything else you need along the way. This program is easy to follow, and it doesn't require any previous experience or knowledge of wellness practices.

What if I don't see myself as a health nut? Is this right for me?

Reclaiming wellness is especially for anyone who feels like the modern wellness community doesn't speak to them. You don't have to "become" a different person to do this program, nor will it turn you into someone else. These wellness practices are part of everyone's ancestry, our DNA, and they help us reclaim our natural, ancestral state of wellness. This is for anyone who is ready to eat healthy, reduce stress, and renew, recharge, and reset their body, mind, and soul.

How will this program help me lose weight?

This is the quintessential question when it comes to health and wellness. *Reclaiming Wellness* is not a diet book, but it does include quite a bit of information on the best, healthiest foods. In addition, weight loss doesn't happen the same way for everyone. It depends on the individual's genetics, hormonal balance history, metabolism, fluid balance, and exercise regimen. Being overweight can also be tied to emotions. It is a complex problem. That said, adopting a more plant-based diet, as this book recommends, will help reduce toxicity in the body, improve metabolism, reduce stress, and eventually, lose weight. Remember, lasting change takes time, and healthy eating is no exception. If you stick to it, you will see results.

Is this program safe for someone who has a preexisting medical condition?

If you have a specific condition or medical concern, I recommend that you consult your doctor before making any changes to your diet or current wellness routine. Most of the practices in this book are safe for most people, but consult with your healthcare provider before you start. They can help you decide which wellness changes will be best for you.

Is this program safe for women who are pregnant or breastfeeding?

Pregnancy is not the ideal time to start a new dietary regime or make drastic changes in lifestyle — other than preparing for the baby's arrival. Of course, all pregnant women should embrace a nutritionally balanced diet, manage stress, and connect with their true self, so many of these practices should be safe during pregnancy. However, as always, if you have medical concerns, please check with your healthcare provider before making changes or starting something new. The same advice applies if you are breastfeeding.

How expensive is all this? I'm on a tight budget.

Reclaiming Wellness is specifically designed for all people regardless of financial situation. Many practices are free; the only cost is time and energy. Other practices require spending money, but how much depends on the individual. For instance, you can do yoga for free at home or spend money to take classes, and classes can range from inexpensive to really pricey. Remember, you are investing in your health and well-being...and you are worth it! Here's another way to think about it: We can pay more up front for fresh produce and yoga classes, or pay more later in the form of poor health and medical bills. It's an easy choice when we put it like this, right?

What if my current work schedule is very strict? How can I make time for all this?

As I say, this program is designed to be flexible to fit your current life, and the rest of this chapter discusses how to incorporate these practices gradually into your existing routine. Don't jump in and try to do everything at once. Following this method, do what's most important to you first, and in whatever ways you can manage. This helps you build long-lasting habits without the stress. If you can't do the full twenty-one-day plan outlined in chapter 10, that's OK. Whatever changes you make will benefit your life and improve wellness.

What if I already lead a pretty healthy lifestyle? Is this only for people who don't?

Few of us lead such healthy lives that we can't improve, but if you're already doing all seven wellness practices, and feel happy and satisfied, then you have already reclaimed your wellness! That said, I always encourage people to kick it up a notch or simply add more weapons to their wellness arsenal. Use this book's method to add any practices that you haven't already explored. Adapt and adjust to make these practices yours.

What if I feel out of place at wellness events and classes? I'm often the only person of color.

I have written this book to help address the diversity and inclusion problem in modern wellness. As I highlight throughout, all modern practices have roots in ancient cultures from around the world, and I hope that all people of color will feel empowered to explore, embrace, and reclaim them. But if you worry about being the only person of color in a class or event, don't go alone! Share this book with friends and family, get them excited about trying these practices, and ask them to join you! In addition, doing a little research may unearth multicultural groups and resources offering these practices in your community.

Preparation and Planning

As I say, we are all busy. Our lives are already packed. We have jobs, families, and community obligations. We have people who depend on us: babies, toddlers, and teenagers; partners and spouses; coworkers and bosses; parents, grandparents, extended family, and friends. We are already doing the best we can to take care of everyone and everything around us and still eat a hot dinner and get a decent night's sleep (if we're lucky). We're frequently stressed and anxious, and while we know we could and want to do better, we often don't know how to make that happen.

The details are different for everyone, but the above scenario is not uncommon. We live full lives, with long to-do lists, lots of plans and goals, and not enough hours in the day to get it all done. We recognize the many blessings in our lives, and yet we can struggle to feel content and at peace on a day-to-day basis. We might wonder if that's even possible, or if achieving it will cost too much in time, energy, and money. We may even have tried several times to do something new and practice self-care in more meaningful ways, but those efforts have fizzled out.

If this describes you, my hope is that, using this method, this time will be different. Preparation is the critical first step. This involves several interrelated activities: cleansing your kitchen to start detoxing your diet; taking inventory of your available space and time; clarifying your intentions; and making a plan for integrating new wellness practices into your life.

In themselves, these activities take time. Some might go more quickly than others, and they don't need to be done in any particular order. However, by focusing on them first, they will allow you to physically, environmentally, and emotionally plan for and embrace the new changes that you are about to reclaim, which will enrich your life for years to come.

The Kitchen Cleanse: Detox Your Diet

Healthier living starts with healthier eating, so before starting a new wellness routine, do a kitchen cleanse. How many times have you walked into your kitchen after a particularly trying day, opened the freezer, and grabbed some ice cream or a frozen pizza? Then later, you feel miserable because, not only did the food not support your wellness, but you had promised to cut back on refined sugars and processed foods, only to give up at the first test of willpower! Trust me, this happens to everyone! To fuel a healthy life, we need healthy fuel, but it is almost impossible to remain disciplined about this — in the face of the many challenges we face every single day — if we don't cleanse and prepare our kitchen to give ourselves a fighting chance.

Yes, we have free will and make our own choices, but what if we help our free will just a little bit? If the only foods in the refrigerator are fruits and healthy snacks, then even if we still end up stress eating, our options will be healthier, and so the consequences will be healthier, too. Using the reduce and replace method, start by filling your kitchen with stuff that will help you ensure a successful wellness journey.

- Make a list of at least ten healthy plant-based snacks, including six or seven you already know and love and three or four that are new to you. Things like guacamole, hummus, celery sticks, apples, berries, bananas, almonds, dairy-free dark chocolate, dates, and frozen edamame are great options.
- When grocery shopping and meal planning, focus on fruits and vegetables. I personally love choosing ingredients that remind me of my childhood and my roots. Things like yucca, sweet plantains, mangoes, and guavas.
- If you have the time and love to cook, you can mix and match and create little snack recipes (like cacao energy balls) as superfood snacks.
- Go through your pantry and refrigerator and get rid of any processed foods full of manufactured or unnatural ingredients. Replace them with healthier options.
- Replace sugary drinks, especially sodas, which have empty calories and little to no nutritional value, with sugar-free alternatives. Or create your own fruit-infused water and store it in large jars in the fridge.

- Look outside the kitchen as well. Review any stashes of snacks and food in your car, at work, or in your gym bag. Reduce and replace to ensure that wherever you go, only healthy food options are available.
- As part of the kitchen cleanse, review your cleaning products. Reduce and replace those with harsh chemicals in favor of others with cleaner, less-harmful ingredients.

Take Inventory of Your Environment

Where and when will you incorporate your new wellness practices? Take inventory of your environment, which includes your schedule, and look for ways to reclaim your space and time.

Reclaim Your Space

Walk around your home and/or office space with an architect's mindset. Is there a room, den, corner, or space that doesn't get a lot of traffic or that other folks don't use? Maybe it doesn't look appealing right now, but could you clean it up and clear it out in order to turn it into your own mini-sanctuary? Sometimes adding a partition or curtain is a simple way to divide a space that's used for several purposes.

Unless you live alone, creating a quiet space might involve coordinating with other family members or roommates. You might already struggle to have any *alone time*. Is there a specific time when the house is quiet enough that you can close the bathroom door and claim that space as yours? If so, what will it take for you to reclaim that space? Do you need to shift your schedule and routine to give yourself that gift? Or is there some other place you might go — such as a park or public space — that you could use for what you need?

Reclaiming your space might require a little juggling and strategizing, but don't despair. It can be done.

Reclaim Your Time

Time is our most precious commodity. A lack of time is the one thing people often cite to me as the reason they can't start or stick with self-care wellness practices. So, it's paramount to review your schedule to figure out when you will accomplish your new wellness routine.

Ideally, pick days and times that are already less busy or less stressful overall. For most people, that means weekends, which is fine unless weekends are also packed and chaotic. However, you also want to practice some wellness every day, so you might need to adjust your current schedule, or create a more structured one, in order to allow for this. Common times of day that tend to work best are first thing in the morning, last thing before bed, and sometimes at lunchtime.

Clarify Intentions and Make Plans

The most important part of preparation is cleansing your mind and emotions and clarifying your intentions. This often means releasing our emotional attachment to our current routine. We can be very attached to the way things are, even when the way things are hasn't truly worked for a while and we are only holding on by a thread. We also have to recognize and address any resistance to change itself; if you need a reminder of the common issues, see "FAQ: Is Reclaiming Wellness for Me?" (pages 150–54). Be honest with yourself and work on purging any emotional blockages and get your mind and soul ready for the bounty that awaits.

Reclaim Your Why

What can help the most is to clarify your intentions. What is your biggest motivating factor? Why are you interested in embracing more wellness practices? Journal your answers. Be specific about the practical details — the what, when, where, and how. Most of all, explore why. Ask yourself, "Why do I want to change? What will wellness do for me?" Explore your emotions, name your values. By answering these questions and getting a clearer picture of why you want to change, you will strengthen your motivation and resolve to achieve those things.

Ask for Assistance

Once you have a clear sense of what you want to accomplish and what you need — in terms of time and space — sit down with the people you live with and let them know that you will be making some changes to practice self-care. At minimum, you want the people who share your home to know what you are doing, even if all you're asking is for them to respect and support your efforts. On the other hand, if you need specific help from certain people, ask for it.

Asking for help can be especially hard for women. By nature or cultural expectation, they often consider themselves caregivers, and they can feel uncomfortable taking time for themselves. Women sometimes forget that the act of receiving is as generous as giving. Mothers may feel that it's "selfish" to do something for themselves, as if this is a comment on their love for or desire to spend quality time with their kids. Ultimately, for those with families, this is another important reason to speak to everyone else in the household. This ensures that everyone knows what you are doing and has a chance to share their feelings and any concerns. And if there are practical issues — such as arranging care or transportation for children at certain times of day, and so on — these can be figured out up front.

Make a Plan

Ultimately, all this preparation leads to creating a specific plan of action for each day or each week. If you live with others, this plan might require some negotiation, and it will certainly change over time. But don't start without one. Remember those wise words: *Fail to plan, plan to fail.* Make sure this plan is easy to follow and detailed: Specify the day, time, and duration of every practice. That way, you can plan everything else in your day, and rinse and repeat that wellness practice with ease. The goal is to never feel like any wellness practice is a burden. Instead, ideally, it will always be a release and a replenishing experience.

A Daily Plan: Easy

What might such a wellness plan look like? The rest of this chapter presents three scenarios: two daily plans and a weekly plan. Then, chapter 10 presents a twenty-one-day plan. However, I don't intend for you to follow these plans exactly. They are meant as examples. They represent various ways someone might use the reduce and replace method to incorporate new wellness practices into their lives. They are practical guides you should adapt to your own needs, but I hope they provide inspiration and encouragement and show you what's possible.

This first one-day plan is "easy." It focuses on incorporating activities from two wellness practices: reclaiming the use of herbs and grounding. For all the plans, I break down each day into three parts (morning, afternoon, and evening), and for the daily plans, I've added some approximate times to simulate what an actual day might look like. However, as I say, adapt these to your own schedule and life, and if you make a plan and one day miss a goal or two, don't stress. Just try not to miss those goals the next day, and if you find you consistently miss certain goals, adjust your schedule or expectations.

Morning

6-8 a.m.: Wake up, eat breakfast, and prepare for the day.

8:30 a.m.: Heat three to four cups of water to make a fennel-ginger tea blend, which optimizes digestion. Put the steeped tea blend in a to-go bottle to take with you and drink through the morning, up to and through lunch. Bring a bag of ashwagandha tea for your afternoon drink.

Afternoon

1 p.m.: During lunch, take a walk outside; find a small park or patch of grass. Take your shoes off and literally walk in the grass for ten to fifteen minutes. Stay longer if possible.

2 p.m.: Make a cup of ashwagandha stress relief tea. After steeping, you can turn it into iced tea and sweeten with a little maple syrup, if you prefer.

4:30 p.m.: If your energy flags in the late afternoon, drink another cup of ashwagandha stress relief tea.

Evening

6:30 p.m.: After getting home from work, change into comfortable clothes and spend half an hour outside. Play with the kids or take a walk with your partner. If the weather permits, go barefoot.

7-9 p.m.: Have dinner and enjoy your evening routine.

9:30 p.m.: Steep a cup of ginger or Tulsi tea to help you relax before having a restorative, good night's sleep.

A Daily Plan: Moderate

Once you start a routine, follow it for at least a week, if not several weeks, before changing it. Wait until it feels natural and you're ready for more. However, if the easy plan seems too easy, great! Take it up a notch. Here is a moderate daily plan that adds practices from two more wellness areas: meditation and movement. Again, remember, the suggested schedule is flexible. If you prefer to move in the morning and meditate before bed, do that.

Morning

6 a.m.: After waking up, do a fifteen-minute meditation. If you wish, use a guided meditation app or practice self-hypnosis instead.
6:30–8 a.m.: Dress, eat breakfast, and prepare for the day.
8:30 a.m.: Heat three to four cups of water to make a fennel-ginger tea blend. Put the steeped tea blend in a to-go bottle, and drink through the morning, up to and through lunch. Bring a bag of ashwagandha tea for your afternoon drink.

Afternoon

1 p.m.: During lunch, take a walk outside in a small park or patch of grass. Take your shoes off and walk barefoot in the grass for ten to fifteen minutes.
2 p.m.: Make a cup of ashwagandha stress relief tea. Turn it into iced tea and sweeten with a little maple syrup, if you prefer.
4:30 p.m.: If your energy flags, drink another cup of ashwagandha stress relief tea.

Evening

6:30 p.m.: After getting home from work, change into workout clothes and exercise for at least thirty minutes. Ideally, if weather permits, do this outside. Run around with your kids in the yard, or follow a workout app or YouTube video. Shake your booty and dance with your partner, but break a sweat. If you have an extra ten minutes, go barefoot in the grass.
7:30–9 p.m.: Eat dinner and enjoy your evening routine.
9:30 p.m.: Steep a cup of ginger or Tulsi tea to help you relax before having a restorative, good night's sleep.

A Weekly Plan: All Seven Practices

Ultimately, however long it takes, the goal is to incorporate all seven practices over the course of a week. Here's what one full week might look like. In this scenario, all practices are included, but some are done every day and some only a few days a week. Realistically, few people have time to do it all every single day.

MONDAY

Morning

Practice meditation or self-hypnosis in a quiet space.
Steep an herbal tea for the day or take supplements with breakfast.
Breakfast is 100% plant-based.

Afternoon

Take a walk for lunch, enjoying the fresh air and walking barefoot in the grass.
Listen to healing sounds or energizing music.
Lunch is 100% plant-based.
Drink an invigorating iced tea.

Evening

After work, exercise or do yoga for thirty minutes.
Dinner is 100% plant-based.
Drink herbal tea to relax in the evening.

TUESDAY

Morning

Practice meditation or self-hypnosis in a quiet space.
Steep herbal tea for the day or take supplements with breakfast.

Afternoon

Drink an invigorating iced or warm herbal tea.

Evening

After work, take a walk, enjoying the fresh air and walking barefoot in the grass.

WEDNESDAY

Morning

Practice meditation or self-hypnosis in a quiet space.
Steep herbal tea for the day or take supplements with breakfast.
Breakfast is 100% plant-based.

Afternoon

Take a walk for lunch, enjoying the fresh air and walking barefoot in the grass.
Listen to healing sounds or energizing music.
Lunch is 100% plant-based.
Drink an invigorating iced tea.

Evening

After work, exercise or do yoga for thirty minutes.
Dinner is 100% plant-based.
Drink herbal tea to relax in the evening.

THURSDAY

Morning

Practice meditation or self-hypnosis in a quiet space.
Steep herbal tea for the day or take supplements with breakfast.

Afternoon

Drink an invigorating iced or warm herbal tea.

Evening

After work, take a walk, enjoying time with others and walking barefoot in the grass.

FRIDAY

Morning

Practice meditation or self-hypnosis in a quiet space.
Steep herbal tea for the day or take supplements with breakfast.
Breakfast is 100% plant-based.

Afternoon

Take a walk for lunch, enjoying the fresh air and walking barefoot in the grass.
Lunch is 100% plant-based.
Drink an invigorating iced tea.

Evening

After work, exercise or do yoga for thirty minutes.
Dinner is 100% plant-based.
Drink herbal tea to relax in the evening.

SATURDAY

Morning

Practice meditation or self-hypnosis in a quiet space.
Steep herbal tea for the day or take supplements with breakfast.
Build a meal plan for the next week and shop for groceries.

Afternoon

Take a walk for lunch, enjoying the fresh air and walking barefoot in the grass.
Engage in a social, community-based activity of any kind; practice ubuntu in all interactions.
Listen to healing sounds or energizing music.
Drink an invigorating iced tea.

Evening

Before dinner, exercise or do yoga for thirty minutes.
Take a relaxing bath with your favorite aromatherapy oils.
Massage your entire body with a relaxing oil-based moisturizer. Drink herbal tea to relax in the evening.

SUNDAY

Morning

Practice meditation or self-hypnosis in a quiet space.
Steep herbal tea for the day or take supplements with breakfast.
Cook three to four plant-based dishes for the week; store them in the refrigerator or freezer.

Afternoon

Do an outdoor activity, enjoying the fresh air and walking barefoot.
Engage in a social, community-based activity; practice ubuntu in all interactions.
Lunch is 100% plant-based.
Drink an invigorating iced tea.

Evening

Take a hot shower, and enjoy the shower steam for several minutes
 afterward.
Dinner is 100% plant-based.
Drink herbal tea to relax in the evening.

10

Recipe for Success

Finally, for an example of what this whole wellness journey might look like, here is a twenty-one-day Reclaiming Wellness plan. This includes all seven wellness practices and many of the individual tools, tips, and strategies I suggest throughout this book. Is this the first thing you should attempt when adopting a wellness plan? No, but this is what you might aim for when you're ready for a challenge.

I hesitate to use the word *challenge* because it implies a struggle or a competition. While this process take times and effort, I've designed it so that hopefully it is never a struggle. Ideally, you'll experience it as a realization, a reawakening of the innate knowledge within. I hope it empowers you to reclaim your well-deserved state of wellness.

It is also important to note that this is not a competition. You are not competing against anyone, especially not with yourself. I encourage you to approach it like this: You are easing your way back to your roots, enjoying every step of the way and becoming healthier, stronger, and happier in the process. If any resistance comes up, or you feel like the process is wearing you down, follow your intuition, ease up for a while, shake your booty, and recommit.

And of course, if you need a bit more support, come find me on the interwebs. See this book's About the Author page for the various places you can find me and reach out online (such as at www.jovankaciares.com).

I hope that each and every one of these practices quite literally fills your life with goodness. I know from experience they can enrich your life to the fullest, without being overwhelming. With time, practice, and patience, you'll find your groove and create your own routine while feeling proud of reclaiming these wellness practices, which have been part of our ancestry for generations. Let's do this!

A Twenty-One-Day Reclaiming Wellness Plan

As I discuss in "Preparation and Planning" (see pages 154–60), you should dedicate adequate time, at least a couple of days, for preparing and planning for this twenty-one-day journey. I've summarized this below (with the assumption that day 1 will be a Monday), but in essence, do whatever you need to do — shop, cook, download apps, get help, sign up for classes, and make appointments — before starting.

One new wrinkle here: I've started each day with an affirmation. This is what I do with my own plans. You can use the affirmations I provide, or replace them with your own affirmation, mantra, or prayer.

Preparation

- Cleanse your kitchen.
- Prepare your space and schedule.

- Build your meal plan and shop for groceries.
- Cook three to four plant-based dishes ahead of time, and store them in the refrigerator or freezer.
- Speak to friends and family members to let them know you are making changes for wellness and would appreciate their support.

WEEK 1
DAY 1

Affirmation

Wellness and happiness are my birthright. I reclaim them and accept them with gratitude.

Morning

In a quiet space, do a ten-minute guided meditation. If you wish, meditate to music.
Steep herbal tea for the day or take supplements with breakfast.
Make a plant-based breakfast, like oatmeal or a green smoothie.

Afternoon

Listen to healing sounds or energizing music.
During lunch, walk outside, ideally barefoot in the grass, for fifteen minutes.
Lunch is 80% plant-based.
Drink an invigorating cup of herbal tea (iced or hot).

Evening

Do thirty minutes of relaxing, stress-reducing tai chi or yoga.
Dinner is 80% plant-based. Suggestion: a Mexican bowl with rice, beans, roasted veggies, and guacamole.
Drink herbal tea to relax.

DAY 2

Affirmation

I feel joy and contentment at this moment, and it stays with me throughout my day.

Morning

In a quiet space, do a ten-minute guided meditation.
Steep herbal tea for the day or take supplements with breakfast.
Breakfast should include plant food: smoothies, oatmeal, chia pudding, whole-wheat toast.

Afternoon

Drink an invigorating iced or warm herbal tea.
Lunch is 80% plant-based. Suggestion: falafel wrap with hummus.

Evening

After work, walk barefoot in the grass, ideally with the kiddos or your partner.
Dinner is 80% plant-based. Suggestion: pasta pesto primavera.

DAY 3

Affirmation

I give myself the care and attention that I deserve.

Morning

In a quiet space, do a ten-minute guided meditation.
Steep herbal tea for the day or take supplements with breakfast.
Make a plant-based breakfast, like oatmeal or a green smoothie.

Afternoon

Listen to healing sounds or energizing music.
During lunch, walk barefoot in a park for fifteen minutes.
Lunch is 80% plant-based. Suggestion: Indian masala with basmati rice.
Drink an invigorating cup of herbal tea, iced or hot.

Evening

Do thirty to sixty minutes of yoga.
Dinner is 80% plant-based. Suggestion: Peruvian quinoa vegetable soup.
Drink herbal tea to relax.

DAY 4

Affirmation

I learn valuable lessons for myself and those I love every single day.

Morning

In a quiet space, do a ten-minute guided meditation.
Steep herbal tea for the day or take supplements with breakfast.
Breakfast should include plant food.

Afternoon

Engage in a social, community-based activity, ideally focused on
    improving the world.
Drink an invigorating iced or warm herbal tea.
Lunch is 80% plant-based. Suggestion: Japanese bento box.

Evening

Take care of indoor plants or an outdoor garden. Touch and talk to the
    plants, and include the kiddos or your partner.
Dinner is 80% plant-based. Suggestion: Vietnamese pho soup.

DAY 5

Affirmation

I am creatively inspired by the world around me.

Morning

In a quiet space, do a ten-minute guided meditation.
Steep herbal tea for the day or take supplements with breakfast.
Make a plant-based breakfast, like oatmeal or a green smoothie.

Afternoon

Listen to healing sounds or energizing music.
During lunch, walk barefoot in a park for fifteen minutes.
Lunch is 80% plant-based. Suggestion: vegetarian paella.
Drink an invigorating cup of herbal tea, iced or hot.

Evening

Do thirty to sixty minutes of yoga.
Dinner is 80% plant-based. Suggestion: Turkish lentil soup.
Drink herbal tea to relax.

DAY 6

Affirmation

I make a difference in the world; my life and work are valuable.

Morning

In a quiet space, do a ten-minute meditation or self-hypnosis practice.
Steep herbal tea for the day or take supplements with breakfast.
Build your meal plan and shop for groceries.
Breakfast should include plant food.

Afternoon

Engage in a social, community-based activity, ideally focused on
    improving the world.
Drink an invigorating iced or warm herbal tea.
Lunch is 80% plant-based. Suggestion: Ethiopian platter with injera.
Listen to healing sounds or energizing music.

Evening

Exercise for thirty minutes, doing any form of movement.
Take a relaxing bath with your favorite aromatherapy oils.
Massage your entire body with a relaxing oil-based moisturizer.
Dinner is 80% plant-based. Suggestion: noodle miso soup.
Drink herbal tea to relax.

DAY 7

Affirmation

I am capable of attracting daily abundance.

Morning

In a quiet space, do a ten-minute meditation or self-hypnosis practice.
Steep herbal tea for the day or take supplements with breakfast.
Cook five to six plant-based dishes for the week; store them in the
   refrigerator or freezer.

Afternoon

Do an outdoor activity, enjoying the fresh air and walking barefoot in
   the grass.
Spend time with others, family or friends; practice ubuntu in all
   interactions.
Listen to healing sounds or energizing music.
Lunch is 80% plant-based. Suggestion: Mexican tamales with side salad.
Drink an invigorating iced tea.

Evening

Take a hot shower, and enjoy the shower steam for several minutes
   afterward.
Dinner is 80% plant-based. Suggestion: vegetable pad Thai.
Drink herbal tea to relax.

WEEK 2

DAY 8

Affirmation

I attract endless prosperity with a positive attitude and an open heart.

Morning

In a quiet space, do a fifteen-minute self-hypnosis practice.
Steep herbal tea for the day or take supplements with breakfast.
Make a plant-based breakfast, like oatmeal or a green smoothie.

Afternoon

Listen to healing sounds or energizing music.
During lunch, walk barefoot in a park for fifteen minutes.
Lunch is 80% plant-based. Suggestion: African jollof rice.
Drink an invigorating cup of herbal tea, iced or hot.

Evening

Do thirty minutes of relaxing, stress-reducing tai chi or yoga.
Dinner is 80% plant-based. Suggestion: Portuguese caldo verde.
Drink herbal tea to relax.

DAY 9

Affirmation

My body is a temple and I am grateful for my ability to heal.

Morning

In a quiet space, do a fifteen-minute self-hypnosis practice.
Steep herbal tea for the day or take supplements with breakfast.
Breakfast should include plant food.

Afternoon

Drink an invigorating iced or warm herbal tea.
Lunch is 80% plant-based. Suggestion: Chinese wonton soup.

Evening

After work, walk barefoot in the grass; ideally, include the kiddos or
    your partner.
Dinner is 80% plant-based. Suggestion: mushroom sauté with mashed
    potatoes.

DAY 10

Affirmation

I am connected with myself at deeper levels to achieve all that I wish for.

Morning

In a quiet space, do a fifteen-minute self-hypnosis practice.
Steep herbal tea for the day or take supplements with breakfast.
Make a plant-based breakfast, like oatmeal or a green smoothie.

Afternoon

Listen to healing sounds or energizing music.
During lunch, walk barefoot in a park for fifteen minutes.
Lunch is 80% plant-based. Suggestion: Japanese soba noodles with
    veggies.
Drink an invigorating cup of herbal tea, iced or hot.

Evening

Do thirty to sixty minutes of yoga.
Dinner is 80% plant-based. Suggestion: Croatian veggie brodetto.
Drink herbal tea to relax.

DAY 11

Affirmation

My daily actions take me closer to my greater purpose.

Morning

In a quiet space, do a fifteen-minute self-hypnosis practice.
Steep herbal tea for the day or take supplements with breakfast.
Breakfast should include plant food.

Afternoon

Engage in a social, community-based activity, ideally focused on
    improving the world.
Drink an invigorating iced or warm herbal tea.
Lunch is 80% plant-based. Suggestion: Indian biryani.

Evening

Take care of indoor plants or an outdoor garden. Touch and talk to the
    plants, and include the kiddos or your partner.
Dinner is 80% plant-based. Suggestion: veggie burger.

DAY 12

Affirmation

*I have all the tools I need to be healthier and happier with each passing
day.*

Morning

In a quiet space, do a fifteen-minute self-hypnosis practice.
Steep herbal tea for the day or take supplements with breakfast.
Make a plant-based breakfast, like oatmeal or a green smoothie.

Afternoon

Listen to healing sounds or energizing music.
During lunch, walk barefoot in a park for fifteen minutes.
Lunch is 80% plant-based. Suggestion: crunchy peanut Thai salad with
avocado.
Drink an invigorating cup of herbal tea, iced or hot.

Evening

Do thirty to sixty minutes of yoga or other exercise.
Dinner is 80% plant-based. Suggestion: vegetable-stuffed Venezuelan
arepas.
Drink herbal tea to relax.

DAY 13

Affirmation

*I feel stronger and more accountable for my spiritual growth with each
passing day.*

Morning

In a quiet space, do a fifteen-minute self-hypnosis practice.
Steep herbal tea for the day or take supplements with breakfast.
Build your meal plan and shop for groceries.
Breakfast should include plant food.

Afternoon

Engage in a social, community-based activity, ideally focused on
improving the world.

Drink an invigorating iced or warm herbal tea.

Lunch is 80% plant-based. Suggestion: Caribbean rice and beans with
sweet plantains.

Listen to healing sounds or energizing music.

Evening

Do thirty to sixty minutes of yoga or other exercise.

Take a relaxing bath with your favorite aromatherapy oils.

Massage your entire body with a relaxing oil-based moisturizer.

Dinner is 80% plant-based. Suggestion: veggie tacos.

Drink herbal tea to relax.

DAY 14

Affirmation

I am enthusiastic about embracing new ways of experiencing joy today.

Morning

In a quiet space, do a fifteen-minute self-hypnosis practice.

Steep herbal tea for the day or take supplements with breakfast.

Cook five to six plant-based dishes for the week; store them in the
refrigerator or freezer.

Afternoon

Do an outdoor activity, enjoying the fresh air and walking barefoot in
the grass.

Spend time with others, family or friends; practice ubuntu in all
interactions.

Listen to healing sounds or energizing music.

Lunch is 80% plant-based. Suggestion: Polish pierogies.

Drink an invigorating iced tea.

Evening

Take a hot shower, and enjoy the shower steam for several minutes afterward.

Dinner is 80% plant-based. Suggestion: Trinidadian pelau-stuffed peppers.

Drink herbal tea to relax.

WEEK 3

DAY 15

Affirmation

My blessings multiply as I share more of myself to serve humanity.

Morning

In a quiet space, do a twenty-minute self-hypnosis practice.

Steep herbal tea for the day or take supplements with breakfast.

Make a plant-based breakfast, like oatmeal or a green smoothie.

Afternoon

Listen to healing sounds or energizing music.

During lunch, walk barefoot in a park for fifteen minutes.

Lunch is 100% plant-based. Suggestion: Thai red curry with rice.

Drink an invigorating cup of herbal tea, iced or hot.

Evening

Do thirty minutes of relaxing, stress-reducing tai chi or yoga.

Dinner is 100% plant-based. Suggestion: ratatouille.

Drink herbal tea to relax.

DAY 16

Affirmation

I let go of fear and doubt and replace them with peace, simplicity, and light.

Morning

In a quiet space, do a twenty-minute self-hypnosis practice.

Steep herbal tea for the day or take supplements with breakfast.

Breakfast should include plant food.

Afternoon

Drink an invigorating iced or warm herbal tea.
Lunch is 80% plant-based. Suggestion: grilled Greek salad with baba ghanoush.

Evening

After work, walk barefoot in the grass, enjoying the fresh air; ideally, include the kiddos or your partner.
Dinner is 80% plant-based. Suggestion: vegan lasagna.

DAY 17

Affirmation

I nourish my body with nutritious foods and my soul with positive thoughts.

Morning

In a quiet space, do a twenty-minute self-hypnosis practice.
Steep herbal tea for the day or take supplements with breakfast.
Make a plant-based breakfast, like oatmeal or a green smoothie.

Afternoon

Listen to healing sounds or energizing music.
During lunch, walk barefoot in a park for fifteen minutes.
Lunch is 100% plant-based. Suggestion: vegetable sushi.
Drink an invigorating cup of herbal tea, iced or hot.

Evening

Do thirty to sixty minutes of yoga.
Dinner is 100% plant-based. Suggestion: vegetarian African peanut soup.
Drink herbal tea to relax.

DAY 18

Affirmation

I happily and easily choose balance in my life for my mind, body, and soul.

Morning

In a quiet space, do a twenty-minute self-hypnosis practice.
Steep herbal tea for the day or take supplements with breakfast.
Breakfast should include plant food.

Afternoon

Engage in a social, community-based activity, ideally focused on
    improving the world.
Drink an invigorating iced or warm herbal tea.
Lunch is 80% plant-based. Suggestion: veggie Buddha bowl.

Evening

Take care of indoor plants or an outdoor garden. Touch and talk to the
    plants, and include the kiddos or your partner.
Dinner is 80% plant-based. Suggestion: Ecuadorian potato soup.

DAY 19

Affirmation

I am liberated from my past and fully present in the here and now.

Morning

In a quiet space, do a twenty-minute self-hypnosis practice.
Steep herbal tea for the day or take supplements with breakfast.
Make a plant-based breakfast, like oatmeal or a green smoothie.

Afternoon

Listen to healing sounds or energizing music.
During lunch, walk barefoot in a park for fifteen minutes.
Lunch is 100% plant-based. Suggestion: mushroom flatbread.
Drink an invigorating cup of herbal tea, iced or hot.

Evening

Do thirty to sixty minutes of yoga or other exercise.
Dinner is 100% plant-based. Suggestion: vegetable lo mein.
Drink herbal tea to relax.

DAY 20

Affirmation

I attract supporting and loving people into my life. We enrich each other's lives, respect each other, and hold each other accountable.

Morning

In a quiet space, do a twenty-minute self-hypnosis practice.
Steep herbal tea for the day or take supplements with breakfast.
Build your meal plan and shop for groceries.
Breakfast should include plant food.

Afternoon

Engage in a social, community-based activity, ideally focused on
    improving the world.
Drink an invigorating iced or warm herbal tea.
Lunch is 80% plant-based. Suggestion: enchiladas with mole sauce.
Listen to healing sounds or energizing music.

Evening

Do thirty to sixty minutes of yoga or other exercise.
Take a relaxing bath with your favorite aromatherapy oils.
Massage your entire body with a relaxing oil-based moisturizer.
Dinner is 80% plant-based. Suggestion: Indian aloo paneer with rice.
Drink herbal tea to relax.

DAY 21

Affirmation

I am the master of my own path; I am proud of who I am.

Morning

In a quiet space, do a twenty-minute self-hypnosis practice.
Steep herbal tea for the day or take supplements with breakfast.
Cook five to six plant-based dishes for the week; store them in the
    refrigerator or freezer.

Afternoon

Do an outdoor activity, enjoying the fresh air and walking barefoot in
    the grass.
Spend time with others, family or friends; practice ubuntu in all
    interactions.
Listen to healing sounds or energizing music.
Lunch is 100% plant-based. Suggestion: Egyptian kushari.
Drink an invigorating iced tea.

Evening

Take a hot shower, and enjoy the shower steam for several minutes
    afterward.
Dinner is 100% plant-based. Suggestion: portobello burger.
Drink herbal tea to relax.

Conclusion

Congratulations! What an awesome journey awaits. Now you are equipped with the knowledge to improve your life and become more empowered with each passing day. I have personally been studying and reclaiming these wellness practices for almost twenty years, and I have found that I'm still learning new and amazing lessons about wellness. I certainly hope this book inspires you to do the same.

Knowledge is a gift. And knowledge coupled with hard work and a positive attitude creates miracles. The practices and traditions described in this book come from humanity's shared culture, from our family and our ancestors. They have been passed down from generation to generation for hundreds and thousands of years. They are your precious legacy and should be preserved — for your own well-being and for the health and wellness of the future generations.

Now, friend, you are one step closer to achieving a state of total wellness. This amazing combination of wellness practices can lead to a healthy lifestyle that creates miracles in your life. I congratulate you and urge you to continue on this path. You're making a positive difference in your life, and your lifestyle changes will create small miracles all over the world. You are reclaiming a life that is whole, peaceful, and successful, and you can share and pass along this gift to others.

Indeed, my hope is that the lessons shared in this book will spread to individuals, groups, and organizations of all kinds, and that we can all help underrepresented communities in the United States and around the world reclaim these wellness practices. If you or your organization are interested in learning more about how you can help, visit www.reclaimingwellnessbook.com for details.

Acknowledgments

I am a woman of many passions, and throughout my life, my parents and two sisters have always been there, curiously offering support, being the best cheerleaders, and believing in me. To my mom and dad, the most loving parents anyone could ask for, thank you for being such stewards of education and knowledge as a way to move up and pay it forward. My older sister, Gisela, one of the wisest people I know, thank you for always offering the best words of encouragement in the precise moment when it's needed most. Marla, arguably the smartest human I've ever met, thank you for being my partner in crime growing up and beyond.

To my life partner, Oscar, the words to express how much you mean to me fall short. You are my rock, my support, my biggest fan, my love. I am a lucky gal to get to love you and be loved by you. Thank you for all the laughter, even in the hardest of times, and for helping me slow down and smell the proverbial roses.

I have been lucky to have had hundreds of teachers, both

educators and curious friends, as well as many professional mentors, present and from afar. My grandparents Mami Eva and Papi Jaime were two of the most curious, smartest people I've ever spoken to. I wish you could have met and chatted with them, but I trust that the stories in this book will help you get to know their wisdom and thirst for knowledge.

Of the many amazing educators, one stands out for her resolve to live her best possible life and give back to the future generation despite insurmountable odds. Ruth Hernández Torres was my first French professor at the University of Puerto Rico. Professor Hernández Torres struggled with breast cancer for years, but that didn't stop her from becoming a powerful community leader, helping create an arts and culture center near the university that still stands today. She reminded her students constantly that the path to achieving our dreams is often filled with struggles that make us wiser and the rewards that much sweeter.

Like Professor Hernández Torres, too many others long before her are gone but never, ever forgotten. I bow to you and honor your work and knowledge with the words in these pages, and I trust they revere your wisdom and the life-changing work you did and passed on to future generations.

I especially want to acknowledge the diseases and conditions that became a catalyst for my healing and new career journey. At twenty-seven or twenty-eight, I was diagnosed with endometriosis and fibroids, one of which was the size of my fist. I also had struggled with irritable bowel syndrome (IBS) and a couple of stomach ulcers. Thanks to the fact that none of these conditions were considered curable by Western medicine, I embarked on a journey where I discovered some of the practices described in this book.

There are several dozen health- and food-related books I read on that journey that are still part of my trusted library. To the authors of these books, thank you for your wisdom and healing words.

To the wonderful experts who contributed their knowledge to this book: vegan chef Jenné Claiborne, hypnotherapist Grace Smith, yoga instructor Melissa Shah, and Ayurvedic practitioner Rita Burgos. Your wisdom and expertise made this book that much richer.

My partner and I started fostering a teenage rescue kitty a few weeks before I started working on this book. King Buddy Kitty (who is now our permanent furry baby) would lie down for hours under the coffee table, keeping me company while I researched and wrote these pages. He was the most amazing company a writer could ever have.

Alongside Buddy Kitty, a daily cup of homemade reishi cacao helped keep me warm, alert, and focused during the long nights of writing.

I have been blessed with incredible friendships throughout my life. From Puerto Rico, my friends Victoria Lorenzo-Kuznick and Yara Meléndez Ordoñez, my college friends (and members of the University of Puerto Rico choir), thank you for over twenty years of friendship, sisterhood, and support throughout this process. I love you both to the moon and back. From New York, my friend Amie Bond, whom I met while working in corporate entertainment and have remained friends with through new cities, new relationships, and trips around the world, thank you for all your support and our pontificating chats about politics and social issues.

Since before I became an entrepreneur, my friend and badass women's advocate Nathalie Molina Niño has been there every single step of the way. Nathalie has, without a doubt, been the most influential person in my entrepreneurial journey, and I know I'm not the only one. To Nathalie, thank you my sister from another mother!

Thank you to my editor, Georgia Hughes, for being so patient and open throughout this whole amazing process and to the entire team at New World Library, for being so flexible and accommodating. Thank you also to my agent, Paul Levine, for putting us all in touch.

To my amazing clients, blog readers, and social media followers, you have taught me so much throughout the years. I am indebted to your wisdom, your vulnerability, and your successes. Every single call, session, class, and post reminds me of why I do this work and how much I love it.

Last but not least, to the communities of color in the United States, Puerto Rico, and around the world, to the ones who will read this book and the ones whose lessons have been passed on for generations. *¡Mil gracias!*

Notes

Chapter 1: Wellness: It's Not Just for the Privileged Few

p. 5   *Americans spend more on healthcare*: The Commonwealth Fund, "U.S. Health Care from a Global Perspective, 2019: Higher Spending, Worse Outcomes," January 20, 2020, https://www.commonwealth fund.org/publications/issue-briefs/2020/jan/us-health-care-global -perspective-2019.

p. 6   *In the United States, approximately 33 percent of adults are overweight*: Cheryl D. Fryar, Margaret D. Carroll, and Cynthia L. Ogden, "Prevalence of Overweight, Obesity, and Extreme Obesity Among Adults Aged 20 and Over: United States, 1960–1962 through 2013–2014," Centers for Disease Control and Prevention, July 18, 2016, https://www.cdc.gov/nchs/data/hestat/obesity_adult_13_14/obesity_adult _13_14.htm.

p. 6   *Heart disease, stroke, and cancer*: Centers for Disease Control and Prevention, "Heart Disease and Stroke," October 7, 2020, https:// www.cdc.gov/chronicdisease/resources/publications/factsheets /heart-disease-stroke.htm; Gary Emerling, "Top 10 Causes of Death in America," *US News*, December 22, 2021, https://www.usnews

.com/news/healthiest-communities/slideshows/top-10-causes-of
-death-in-america?slide=10.

p. 6   *Nearly half (47 percent) of American adults have high blood pressure*: Centers for Disease Control and Prevention, "Facts About Hypertension," September 27, 2021, https://www.cdc.gov/bloodpressure/facts.htm.

p. 6   *About 38 percent of Americans have high cholesterol*: Centers for Disease Control and Prevention, "Cholesterol," September 27, 2021, https://www.cdc.gov/cholesterol/index.htm.

p. 6   *About 80 percent of heart disease–related deaths*: Ryan Jaslow, "CDC: 200,000 Heart Disease Deaths Could Be Prevented Each Year," September 3, 2013, https://www.cbsnews.com/news/cdc-200000-heart -disease-deaths-could-be-prevented-each-year.

p. 6   *50 million people have at least one autoimmune disorder*: American Autoimmune Related Diseases Association, "Autoimmune Facts," brochure, https://www.aarda.org/wp-content/uploads/2019/12/1 -in-5-Brochure.pdf.

p. 6   *one of the lowest life expectancies in the industrialized world*: United Health Foundation, "America's Health Rankings: Comparison with Other Nations, 2016 Annual Report," accessed January 10, 2022, https://www.americashealthrankings.org/learn/reports/2016-annual -report/comparison-with-other-nations; CIA World Factbook, "Country Comparisons: Life Expectancy at Birth," accessed January 10, 2022, https://www.cia.gov/the-world-factbook/field/life-expectancy -at-birth/country-comparison.

Chapter 2: Plants That Help Us Heal

p. 16   *In fact, the World Health Organization estimates*: "WHO Global Report on Traditional and Complementary Medicine: 2019," World Health Organization, 2019, https://www.who.int/traditional -complementary-integrative-medicine/WhoGlobalReportOn TraditionalAndComplementaryMedicine2019.pdf.

p. 19   *To get an expert's perspective on Ayurveda*: Rita Burgos, interview with author, April 20, 2021.

p. 23   *This section features a short list of those botanicals*: The information in these lists is from my own work as an herbalist and from Mohd Sajjad Ahmad Khan, Iqbal Ahmad, and Debprasad Chattopadhyay, *New Look to Phytomedicine* (London: Academic Press, 2018).

p. 31   *The Aztec Empire of Mexico and Central America used*: William Gates, *An Aztec Herbal: The Classic Codex of 1552* (Garden City, NY: Dover Publications, 2000).

Chapter 3: Going Within

p. 37   *Today, medical and scientific research includes hundreds*: Alvin Powell,
"When Science Meets Mindfulness," *Harvard Gazette*, April 9, 2018,
https://news.harvard.edu/gazette/story/2018/04/harvard-researchers
-study-how-mindfulness-may-change-the-brain-in-depressed-patients.

p. 38   *"art of using mental imagery and affirmation"*: Shakti Gawain, *Creative Visualization: Use the Power of Your Imagination to Create What
You Want in Your Life* (1978; repr., Novato, CA: New World Library,
2002), back cover copy.

p. 40   *According to the Mayo Clinic, hypnosis has been*: "Hypnosis," Mayo
Clinic, accessed November 30, 2021, https://www.mayoclinic.org
/tests-procedures/hypnosis/about/pac-20394405.

p. 41   *"In research conducted by Kirsch at Harvard"*: Markham Heid, "Is
Hypnosis Real? Here's What Science Says," *Time*, September 4, 2018,
https://time.com/5380312/is-hypnosis-real-science.

p. 41   *"After listening to a hypnosis recording twice/day"*: Grace Smith,
https://getgrace.com, citing Alfred A. Barrios, "Hypnotherapy: A
Reappraisal," *Psychotherapy: Theory, Research & Practice* 7, no. 1
(spring 1970), 2–7, https://doi.org/10.1037/h0086544.

p. 43   *According to Grace, hypnosis began in ancient Egypt*: The historical
details and quotes in this section are from Grace Smith, interview
with author, April 23, 2021.

Chapter 4: Yoga and Other Forms of Movement

p. 53   *However, according to research at John Hopkins University*: "9 Benefits
of Yoga," John Hopkins Medicine, Health, accessed June 30, 2021,
https://www.hopkinsmedicine.org/health/wellness-and-prevention
/9-benefits-of-yoga.

p. 54   *"It's practicing this ability to direct your mind"*: Melissa Shah, interview with author, April 26, 2021.

p. 61   *According to the World Health Organization, here are some*: "Physical
Inactivity a Leading Cause of Disease and Disability, Warns WHO,"
World Health Organization, April 4, 2002, https://www.who.int
/news/item/04-04-2002-physical-inactivity-a-leading-cause-of
-disease-and-disability-warns-who.

Chapter 5: A Plant-Based Diet

p. 67   *"At this point, any scientist, doctor, journalist, or policy maker"*: T. Colin
Campbell and Howard Jacobson, *Whole: Rethinking the Science of
Nutrition* (Dallas: BenBella Books, 2014), xiii.

p. 68   *"I believe that health is wealth"*: All quotes by Jenné Claiborne from interview with author, April 28, 2021.

p. 69   *A crossover trial, published in February 2021*: Neal D. Barnard et al., "A Mediterranean Diet and Low-Fat Vegan Diet to Improve Body Weight and Cardiometabolic Risk Factors: A Randomized, Crossover Trial," *Journal of the American College of Nutrition* (February 5, 2021), https://pubmed.ncbi.nlm.nih.gov/33544066.

p. 69   *A 2017 review of more than ten studies found*: Michelle McMacken and Sapana Shah, "A Plant-Based Diet for the Prevention and Treatment of Type 2 Diabetes," *Journal of Geriatric Cardiology* 14, no. 5 (May 2017), https://www.ncbi.nlm.nih.gov/pmc/articles /PMC5466941.

p. 70   *A 2019 case study published in the* Permanente Journal: Maximilian A. Storz, "Is There a Lack of Support for Whole-Food, Plant-Based Diets in the Medical Community?" *Permanente Journal* (winter 2019), https://doi.org/10.7812/TPP/18-068.

p. 70   *The Adventist Health Studies, a series of long-term*: Loma Linda University Health, "About Adventist Health Studies," accessed December 8, 2021, https://adventisthealthstudy.org/about.

p. 70   *This population was half as likely to be on medications*: Michael Greger, MD, "Plant Based Diet Can Cut Your Odds of Needing Medication in Half," March 7, 2012, https://www.yahoo.com /lifestyle/tagged/health/green/plant-based-diet-cut-odds-needing -medication-half-202900956.html.

p. 70   *Dr. Kim Williams, an African American cardiologist*: Crystal Phend, "10 Questions: Kim Williams, MD," *MedPage Today*, April 2014, https://www.medpagetoday.com/Cardiology/Prevention/45250.

p. 70   *Since 1978, Dr. Dean Ornish has conducted studies*: "Ornish Lifestyle Medicine: The Proof," accessed January 4, 2022, https://www.ornish .com/undo-it.

p. 70   *In his clinical research, which is described*: Neal Barnard and Bryanna Clark Grogan, *Dr. Neal Barnard's Program for Reversing Diabetes: The Scientifically Proven System for Reversing Diabetes without Drugs* (New York: Rodale, 2007).

p. 76   *Americans consume 0.9 cups of fruit and 1.4 cups of vegetables a day*: Hayden Stewart and Jeffrey Hyman, "Americans Still Can Meet Fruit and Vegetable Dietary Guidelines for $2.10–$2.60 per Day," USDA Economic Research Service, June 2019, https://www.ers.usda.gov /amber-waves/2019/june/americans-still-can-meet-fruit-and -vegetable-dietary-guidelines-for-210-260-per-day.

p. 76   *In the 1980s, scientists compared diets rich*: T. Colin Campbell and
         Thomas M. Campbell, *The China Study: The Most Comprehensive
         Study of Nutrition Ever Conducted and the Startling Implications for
         Diet, Weight Loss and Long-Term Health* (Dallas: BenBella Books,
         2006).

p. 91   *Multiple studies have shown that if we grew crops*: University of
         Minnesota, "Existing Cropland Could Feed Four Billion More by
         Dropping Biofuels and Animal Feed," *ScienceDaily*, August 1, 2013,
         https://www.sciencedaily.com/releases/2013/08/130801125704.htm.

p. 91   *Livestock and their by-products account*: Robert Goodland and Jeff
         Anhang, "Livestock and Climate Change," *World Watch Magazine*,
         November/December 2009.

p. 91   *animal agriculture is responsible for*: Hiroko Tabuchi, Claire Rigby,
         and Jeremy White, "Amazon Deforestation, Once Tamed, Comes
         Roaring Back," *New York Times*, February 24, 2017, https://www
         .nytimes.com/2017/02/24/business/energy-environment/deforestation
         -brazil-bolivia-south-america.html?_r=0.

Chapter 6: Oil, Water, and Heat

p. 95   *Sweating helps burn calories as the body*: Chris Iliades, "Do You Burn
         More Calories in Hot or Cold Temperatures?," Livestrong.com,
         August 30, 2021, https://www.livestrong.com/article/526014-does
         -your-body-burn-more-calories-if-you-are-hot-or-if-you-are-cold.

p. 99   *A Turkish hammam — the word means "spreader of warmth"*: Nina
         Pfuderer, "The Meaning of Hammam in Moroccan Culture," Abury,
         September 13, 2017, https://abury.net/blogs/abury-blog/the-meaning
         -of-hammam-in-moroccan-culture.

Chapter 7: Music and Community

p. 122   *Research has shown that people with stronger social*: Yang Claire
         Yang et al., "Social Relationships and Physiological Determinants of
         Longevity Across the Human Life Span," *Proceedings of the National
         Academy of Sciences* 113, no. 3 (January 2016), https://www.pnas.org
         /content/113/3/578.

p. 122   *A study involving over three hundred thousand people*: "The Health
         Benefits of Strong Relationships," Harvard Health Publishing, De-
         cember 1, 2010, https://www.health.harvard.edu/staying-healthy
         /the-health-benefits-of-strong-relationships.

p. 122   *"the size and quality of a person's social ties"*: Elahe Izadi, "Your Relationships Are Just as Important to Your Health as Diet and Exercise,"
Washington Post, January 5, 2016, https://www.washingtonpost.com
/news/to-your-health/wp/2016/01/05/your-relationships-are-just-as
-important-to-your-health-as-exercising-and-eating-well.

p. 124   *The term is often translated as a phrase*: Fainos Mangena, "Hunhu/
Ubuntu in the Traditional Thought of Southern Africa" Internet
Encyclopedia of Philosophy, accessed June 30, 2021, https://iep.utm
.edu/hunhu.

Chapter 8: Grounding and Nature

p. 139   *Here are some of the most common climate change–related*: Pari-
tosh Kasotia, "The Health Effects of Global Warming: Developing
Countries Are the Most Vulnerable," United Nations, UN Chronicle,
accessed June 30, 2020, https://www.un.org/en/chronicle/article
/health-effects-global-warming-developing-countries-are-most
-vulnerable.

p. 143   *Roughly 40 percent of the food people buy*: Dana Gunders, "Wasted:
How America Is Losing Up to 40 Percent of Its Food from Farm to
Fork to Landfill," Natural Resources Defense Council, August 16,
2017, https://www.nrdc.org/resources/wasted-how-america-losing
-40-percent-its-food-farm-fork-landfill.

Bibliography

Introduction

Egede, Leonard E. "Race, Ethnicity, Culture, and Disparities in Health Care." *Journal of General Internal Medicine* 21, no. 6 (June 2006). https://www.ncbi.nlm.nih.gov/pmc/articles/PMC1924616.

Law, Violet. "Coronavirus Is Disproportionately Killing African Americans." Aljazeera, April 10, 2020. https://www.aljazeera.com/news/2020/4/10/coronavirus-is-disproportionately-killing-african-americans.

Chapter 1: Wellness: It's Not Just for the Privileged Few

Tikkanen, Roosa, and Melinda Abrams. "US Health Care from a Global Perspective, 2019: Higher Spending, Worse Outcomes?" Commonwealth Fund, January 30, 2020. https://www.commonwealthfund.org/publications/issue-briefs/2020/jan/us-health-care-global-perspective-2019.

Chapter 2: Plants That Help Us Heal

Bussmann, Rainer W. "The Globalization of Traditional Medicine in Northern Peru: From Shamanism to Molecules." *Evidence-Based Complementary and Alternative Medicine* (2013). https://www.ncbi.nlm.nih.gov/pmc /articles/PMC3888705.

Gates, William. *An Aztec Herbal: The Classic Codex of 1552.* Garden City, NY: Dover Publications, 2000.

Low Dog, Tieraona. *Healthy at Home: Get Well and Stay Well Without Prescriptions.* Washington, DC: National Geographic, 2014.

Storl, Wolf D. *The Untold History of Healing: Plant Lore and Medicinal Magic from the Stone Age to Present.* New York: Penguin Random House, 2017.

Thomason, Timothy C. "The Role of Altered States of Consciousness in Native American Healing." Northern Arizona University. Accessed June 30, 2020. https://www.cuyamungueinstitute.com/articles-and-news/the-role-of -altered-states-of-consciousness-in-native-american-healing.

Weis-Bohlen, Susan. *Ayurveda Beginner's Guide: Essential Ayurvedic Principles and Practices to Balance and Heal Naturally.* San Antonio, TX: Althea Press, 2018.

Chapter 3: Going Within

Eisler, Melissa. "The History of Meditation." Chopra, July 28, 2014. https:// chopra.com/articles/the-history-of-meditation.

"Hypnosis." Mayo Clinic. Accessed June 30, 2021. https://www.mayoclinic.org /tests-procedures/hypnosis/about/pac-20394405.

Picotte, Tristan. "Storytelling in Native American Cultures." Partnership with Native Americans, October 16, 2018. http://blog.nativepartnership.org /storytelling-in-native-american-cultures.

Powell, Alvin. "When Science Meets Mindfulness." *Harvard Gazette*, April 9, 2018. https://news.harvard.edu/gazette/story/2018/04/harvard-researchers -study-how-mindfulness-may-change-the-brain-in-depressed-patients.

Ross, Ashley. "How Meditation Went Mainstream." *Time*, March 9, 2016. https://time.com/4246928/meditation-history-buddhism.

Spiegel, D., and J. R. Bloom. "Group Therapy and Hypnosis Reduce Metastatic Breast Carcinoma Pain." *Psychosomatic Medicine* 45, no. 4 (August 1983). https://pubmed.ncbi.nlm.nih.gov/6622622.

Chapter 4: Yoga and Other Forms of Movement

Basavaraddi, Ishwar. "Yoga: Its Origin, History and Development." Indian Ministry of External Affairs, Public Diplomacy, April 23, 2015. https:// www.mea.gov.in/in-focus-article.htm?25096/Yoga+Its+Origin+History +and+Development.

Freese, Jens et al. "The Sedentary (R)evolution: Have We Lost Our Metabolic Flexibility?" *F1000 Research*, February 2, 2018. https://www.ncbi.nlm.nih .gov/pmc/articles/PMC5710317.

Jagim, Andrew. "The Importance of Movement." Mayo Clinic Health System, June 8, 2020. https://www.mayoclinichealthsystem.org/hometown-health /featured-topic/the-importance-of-movement.

Lam, Paul. "History of Tai Chi." Tai Chi for Health Institute, 2007. Accessed June 30, 2021. https://taichiforhealthinstitute.org/history-of-tai-chi-2.

Ortner, Nick. *The Tapping Solution: A Revolutionary System for Stress-Free Living*. Carlsbad, CA: Hay House, 2014.

"A Short History of Yoga in India." Replenish Living. Accessed June 30, 2021. https://www.replenishliving.com/a-short-history-of-yoga-in-india.

Talmon-Chvaicer, Maya. *The Hidden History of Capoeira: A Collision of Cultures in the Brazilian Battle Dance*. Austin: University of Texas Press, 2007.

Venkatraman, Sakshi, "White Women Co-opted Pandemic Yoga. Now, South Asian Instructors Are Taking It Back." NBC News, April 13, 2021. https://www.nbcnews.com/news/asian-america/white-women-co-opted -pandemic-yoga-now-south-asian-instructors-n1263952.

Chapter 5: A Plant-Based Diet

Ali, Rasha. "Meat-Free and Plant-Based Diets Are Gaining Popularity. Here's What You Need to Know." *USA Today*, February 26, 2019. https://www .usatoday.com/story/life/2019/02/26/vegan-vegetarian-pescatarian -flexitarian-plant-based-no-meat-diets-compared/2949993002.

Barnard, Neal D., Jihad Alwarith, Emilie Rembert, Liz Brandon, Minh Nguyen, Andrea Goergen, Taylor Horne et al. "A Mediterranean Diet and Low-Fat Vegan Diet to Improve Body Weight and Cardiometabolic Risk Factors: A Randomized, Cross-over Trial." *Journal of the American College of Nutrition* (February 2021). https://www.tandfonline.com/doi/full/10.1080/0731 5724.2020.1869625.

Bower, Kelly M., Roland J. Thorpe, Jr., Charles Rohde, and Darrell J. Gaskin. "The Intersection of Neighborhood Racial Segregation, Poverty, and Urbanicity and Its Impact on Food Store Availability in the United States." *Preventive Medicine* 58 (January 2014). https://www.ncbi.nlm.nih.gov /pmc/articles/PMC3970577.

Dunn, Rob. "Human Ancestors Were Nearly All Vegetarians." *Scientific American*, July 23, 2012. https://blogs.scientificamerican.com/guest-blog/human -ancestors-were-nearly-all-vegetarians.

Imamura, Fumiaki et al. "Dietary Quality among Men and Women in 187 Countries in 1990 and 2010: A Systematic Assessment." *Lancet Global*

Health 3, no. 3 (March 2015). https://www.thelancet.com/journals/langlo /article/PIIS2214-109X(14)70381-X/fulltext.

"Sample Registration System Baseline Survey 2014." Office of the Registrar General & Census Commissioner, Indian Ministry of Home Affairs. Accessed June 30, 2021. https://www.censusindia.gov.in/vital_statistics /BASELINE%20TABLES07062016.pdf.

Toumpanakis, Anastasios, Triece Turnbull, and Isaura Alba-Barba. "Effectiveness of Plant-Based Diets in Promoting Well-Being in the Management of Type 2 Diabetes: A Systematic Review." *BMJ Open Diabetes Research & Care* (July 2018). https://drc.bmj.com/content/bmjdrc/6/1/e000534.full.pdf.

Tuso, Philip J., Mohamed H. Ismail, Benjamin P. Ha, Carole Bartolotto. "Nutritional Update for Physicians: Plant-Based Diets." *Permanent Journal* 17, no. 2 (spring 2013). https://www.ncbi.nlm.nih.gov/pmc/articles/PMC 3662288.

"Vegan Cuisine Guide: Plant-Based Foods Worldwide." Vegan.com. Accessed June 30, 2021. https://vegan.com/food/cuisines.

Williams, Kim. "CardioBuzz: Vegan Diet, Healthy Heart?" *MedPage Today*, July 21, 2014. https://www.medpagetoday.com/opinion/cardiobuzz/46860.

Chapter 6: Oil, Water, and Heat

Diller, Kenneth R. "Heat Transfer in Health and Healing." *Journal of Heat Transfer* 137, no. 10 (October 2015). https://www.ncbi.nlm.nih.gov/pmc /articles/PMC4462861.

"Essential Oil." *Encyclopedia Britannica*, May 15, 2019. Accessed June 30, 2021. https://www.britannica.com/topic/essential-oil/Chemical-composition.

Lee, Annabelle. "Jjimjilbang: A Microcosm of Korean Leisure Culture." *Korean Herald*, April 1, 2010. http://www.koreaherald.com/view.php?ud =20100331000120.

Sood, Suemedha. "The Origins of Bathhouse Culture Around the World." *BBC News*, Travel, November 29, 2012. https://www.bbc.com/travel/article /20121129-the-origins-of-bathhouse-culture-around-the-world.

Chapter 7: Music and Community

Buettner, Dan. *The Blue Zones: 9 Lessons for Living Longer from the People Who've Lived the Longest.* 2nd ed. Washington, DC: National Geographic, 2012.

Chaudhary, Kulreet. *Sound Medicine: How to Use the Ancient Science of Sound to Heal the Body and Mind.* New York: HarperCollins Publishers, 2020.

"The Health Benefits of Strong Relationships." Harvard Health Publishing, December 1, 2020. https://www.health.harvard.edu/staying-healthy /the-health-benefits-of-strong-relationships.

Izadi, Elahe. "Your Relationships Are just as Important to Your Health as Diet and Exercise." *Washington Post*, January 5, 2016. https://www.washington post.com/news/to-your-health/wp/2016/01/05/your-relationships-are -just-as-important-to-your-health-as-exercising-and-eating-well.

Mangena, Fainos. "Hunhu/Ubuntu in the Traditional Thought of Southern Africa." Internet Encyclopedia of Philosophy. Accessed June 30, 2021. https://iep.utm.edu/hunhu/#H4.

Chapter 8: Grounding and Nature

Chevalier, Gaétan et al. "Earthing: Health Implications of Reconnecting the Human Body to the Earth's Surface Electrons." *Journal of Environmental and Public Health* (January 2012). https://www.ncbi.nlm.nih.gov/pmc /articles/PMC3265077.

"Climate Change and Health." World Health Organization, October 30, 2021. https://www.who.int/news-room/fact-sheets/detail/climate-change-and -health.

"Climate Effects on Health." Centers for Disease Control and Prevention, Climate and Health. Accessed June 30, 2021. https://www.cdc.gov/climate andhealth/effects/default.htm.

"What Is Earthing." Earthing Institute. Accessed June 30, 2021. https:// earthinginstitute.net/what-is-earthing.

Resources and Recommended Reading

The following are helpful resources for finding classes, practitioners, and information in your area. Within each topic, online resources are listed first, followed by books and films. This list is by no means exhaustive, but it should get you started. Enjoy!

Acupuncture / Traditional Chinese Medicine

American Association of Acupuncture and Oriental Medicine, https://www.aaaomonline.org
American Traditional Chinese Medicine Association, https://atcma-us.org
Maciocia, Giovanni. *The Foundations of Chinese Medicine*. London: Elsevier, 2015.
———. *The Practice of Chinese Medicine*. London: Churchill Livingstone, 2007.

Animal Welfare

Scully, Matthew. *Dominion: The Power of Man, the Suffering of Animals, and the Call to Mercy*. New York: St. Martin's Griffin, 2002.

Ayurveda

Association of Ayurvedic Professionals of North America (AAPNA),
  https://www.aapna.org

Ayurvedic Institute, https://www.ayurveda.com/resources/overview

Chopra, Deepak. *Perfect Health*. New York: Three Rivers Press, 1991/2000.

Lad, Vasant. *Ayurveda: The Science of Self-Healing: A Practical Guide*. Twin
  Lakes, WI: Lotus Press, 1984.

———. *The Complete Book of Ayurvedic Home Remedies*. New York: Three
  Rivers Press, 1998.

Weis-Bohlen, Susan. *Ayurveda Beginner's Guide: Essential Ayurvedic Principles*.
  San Antonio, TX: Althea Press, 2018.

Cleansing/Detox

Fitzgerald, Patricia. *The Detox Solution*. Santa Monica, CA: Illumination Press,
  2001.

Jordan, Loree Taylor. *Detox for Life*. Campbell, CA: Madison Publishing, 2002.

Junger, Alejandro. *Clean*. New York: HarperOne, 2009.

Stiles, Tara. *Clean Mind, Clean Body*. New York: Dey Street Books, 2020.

Cookbooks

Claiborne, Jenné. *Sweet Potato Soul*. New York: Harmony Books, 2018.

Derseweh, Nicole, and Whitney Lauritsen. *Vegan Ketogenic Diet Cookbook*.
  Emeryville, CA: Rockridge Press, 2020.

Kenney, Matthew, and Sarma Melngailis. *Raw Food Real World*. New York:
  Regan Books, 2005.

O'Brien, Susan. *The Gluten-Free Vegan*. New York: Marlowe & Company, 2007.

Okamoto, Toni, and Michelle Cehn. *The Friendly Vegan Cookbook*. Dallas:
  BenBella Books, 2020.

Phyo, Ani. *Ani's Raw Food Desserts*. Cambridge, MA: Da Capo Press, 2009.

———. *Ani's Raw Food Kitchen*. New York: Marlowe & Company, 2007.

Pierson, Joy, Bart Potenza, and Barbara Scott-Goodman. *The Candle Cafe
  Cookbook*. New York: Clarkson Potter, 2003.

Pirello, Christina. *This Crazy Vegan Life*. New York: Home, 2008.

Terry, Bryant. *Vegan Soul Kitchen*. Cambridge, MA: Da Capo Press, 2009.

Environment

The Daily Green, https://the-daily-green.com

Earth911, https://earth911.com

Green America, https://www.greenamerica.org
Take a Bite Out of Climate Change, https://www.takeabitecc.org

Farmers Markets

USDA, National Farmers Market Directory, https://www.ams.usda.gov/local
-food-directories/farmersmarkets

Food Co-ops

Co-op Directory Service Listing, http://www.coopdirectory.org/directory.htm
LocalHarvest, https://www.localharvest.org

Grounding/Earthing

Grounded, https://grounded.com
McMorrow, Erin Yu-Juin. *Grounded A Fierce, Feminine Guide to Connecting with the Soil and Healing from the Ground Up.* Boulder, CO: Sounds True, 2021.
Ober, Clinton, Martin Zucker, and Stephen Sinatra. *Earthing: The Most Important Health Discovery Ever!* Laguna Beach, CA: Basic Health Publications, 2014.

Healthy Lifestyle and Diets*

NutritionFacts.org, https://nutritionfacts.org
Physicians Committee for Responsible Medicine, https://www.pcrm.org
T. Colin Campbell Center for Nutrition Studies, https://nutritionstudies.org
Tree of Life Community, https://treeoflife.mn.co
Barnard, Neal, and Bryanna Clark Grogan. *Dr. Neal Barnard's Program for Reversing Diabetes.* New York: Rodale, 2007.
Bittman, Mark. *Food Matters.* New York: Simon & Schuster, 2009.
Campbell, T. Colin, and Thomas M. Campbell. *The China Study.* Dallas: BenBella Books, 2006.
Carr, Kris. *Crazy Sexy Diet.* Guilford, CT: skirt!, 2011.
Case, Shelley, Iona Glabus, and Brian Danchuk. *Gluten-Free Diet.* Regina, Canada: Case Nutrition Consulting, 2001/2010.
Chopra, Deepak. *Perfect Health.* New York: Three Rivers Press, 1991/2000.

---

*   See also "Cookbooks" on p. 202 and "Vegetarian/Vegan Lifestyle" on p. 207.

Clark, Hulda Regehr. *The Cure for All Diseases*. Chula Vista, CA: New Century Press, 1995.

Clement, Brian, and Theresa Foy DiGeronimo. *Living Foods for Optimum Health*. New York: Three Rivers Press, 1996.

Cousens, Gabriel. *Conscious Eating*. Berkeley, CA: North Atlantic Books, 2000.

Diamond, Harvey, and Marilyn Diamond. *Fit For Life*. New York: Warner Books, 1985.

Dries, Jan, and Inge Dries. *Complete Book of Food Combining*. Rockport, MA: Element Books, 1998.

Ehret, Arnold. *Mucusless Diet Healing System*. New York: Benedict Lust Publications, 2018.

Freston, Kathy. *Quantum Wellness*. New York: Weinstein Books, 2008.

Gannon, Sharon. *Yoga and Vegetarianism*. San Rafael, CA: Mandala Publishing, 2008.

Greger, Michael, and Gene Stone. *How Not to Die*. New York: Flatiron Books, 2015.

Lappé, Frances Moore. *Diet for a Small Planet*. New York: Ballantine Books, 1991.

McDougall, John, and Mary McDougall. *The Starch Solution*. New York: Rodale, 2012.

McQuirter, Tracye Lynn. *By Any Greens Necessary*. Chicago: Lawrence Hill Books, 2010.

Ornish, Dean. *Eat More, Weigh Less*. New York: HarperTorch, 1993/2001.

———. *The Spectrum*. New York: Ballantine Books, 2007.

Pollan, Michael. *In Defense of Food*. New York: Penguin Books, 2009.

——— *The Omnivore's Dilemma*. New York: Penguin Books, 2006/2016.

Ritchason, Jack. *The Little Herb Encyclopedia*. Salt Lake City, UT: Woodland Publishing, 1995.

Robbins, John. *Diet for a New America*. Tiburon, CA: H J Kramer / New World Library, 1987/2012.

———. *The Food Revolution*. San Francisco: Conari Press, 2011.

———. *Healthy at 100*. New York: Ballantine Books, 2006.

Tuttle, Will M. *The World Peace Diet*. New York: Lantern Books, 2016.

Vasey, Christopher. *The Acid-Alkaline Diet for Optimum Health*. Rochester, VT: Healing Arts Press, 1999/2006.

Woodham, Anne, and David Peters. *The Encyclopedia of Healing Therapies*. London: Dorling Kindersley, 1997.

Herbal Medicine

American Herbalists Guild, https://www.americanherbalistsguild.com

American Herbal Pharmacopoeia, https://herbal-ahp.org

American Herbal Products Association, https://www.ahpa.org

Chevallier, Andrew. *Encyclopedia of Herbal Medicine*. London: Dorling Kindersley, 1996/2016.

Cunningham, Scott. *Encyclopedia of Magical Herbs*. St. Paul, MN: Llewellyn Publications, 2003.

Gladstar, Rosemary. *Medicinal Herbs*. North Adams, MA: Storey Publishing, 2012.

Hoffmann, David. *Medical Herbalism*. New York: Healing Arts Press, 2003.

Tierra, Michael. *The Way of Herbs*. New York: Pocket Books, 1980/1998.

Wood, Matthew. *The Practice of Traditional Western Herbalism*. Berkeley, CA: North Atlantic Books, 2004.

Holistic Health Practitioners

Academy of Integrative Health & Medicine, https://aihm.org

American Holistic Health Association, http://ahha.org

Hot Springs, Saunas, and Steam Baths

Global Wellness Institute, Hot Springs Initiative Resources, https://globalwellnessinstitute.org/initiatives/hot-springs-initiative /global-hot-springs-resources

Roeder, Giselle. *Sauna: The Hottest Way to Good Health*. Vancouver, Canada: Alive Books, 2002.

Wilson, Lawrence. *Sauna Therapy for Detoxification and Healing*. Prescott, AZ: LD Wilson Consultants, 2016.

Hypnosis

American Association of Professional Hypnotherapists, http://www.aaph.org

American Society of Clinical Hypnosis, https://www.asch.net

Arden, John. *Rewire Your Brain*. Hoboken, NJ: John Wiley & Sons, 2010.

Smith, Grace. *Close Your Eyes, Get Free*. New York: Da Capo Press, 2018.

Weiss, Brian. *Many Lives, Many Masters*. New York: Touchstone, 1988.

Juicing

Meyerowitz, Steve. *Power Juices, Super Drinks: Quick, Delicious Recipes to Prevent & Reverse Disease*. New York: Kensington Publishing, 2000.

Murray, Michael T. *The Complete Book of Juicing*. New York: Clarkson Potter, 2013.

Null, Gary, and Shelly Null. *The Joy of Juicing*. New York: Avery, 1992/2013.
Smith, JJ. *Green Smoothies for Life*. New York: Atria Books, 2016.

Manifesting

Dyer, Wayne. *Manifest Your Destiny*. New York: Harper Perennial, 1998.
———. *The Power of Intention*. Carlsbad, CA: Hay House, 2005.
Gawain, Shakti. *Creative Visualization*. Novato, CA: New World Library, 1978/2002.

Massage

American Massage Therapy Association, https://www.amtamassage.org

Meditation

Allen, Jennie. *Get Out of Your Head*. New York: Waterbrook, 2020.
American Meditation Society, https://www.americanmeditationsociety.org
Harris, Dan, and Jeff Warren. *Meditation for Fidgety Skeptics*. New York: Spiegel & Grau, 2017.
Suzuki, Shunryu. *Zen Mind, Beginner's Mind*. Boston: Shambhala, 2006.

Self-Improvement

Brown, Brené. *Daring Greatly*. New York: Avery, 2012.
Ruiz, don Miguel. *The Four Agreements: A Practical Guide to Personal Freedom*. San Rafael, CA: Amber-Allen Publishing, 2018.
Sincero, Jen. *You Are a Badass*. Philadelphia: Running Press, 2013.
Tolle, Eckhart. *The Power of Now*. Vancouver, Canada: Namaste Publishing, 1999/2004.
Tracy, Brian. *Eat That Frog!*. Oakland, CA: Berrett-Koehler Publishers, 2017.
Vanzant, Iyanla. *Yesterday, I Cried*. New York: Atria, 1999.

Sound Healing

Sound Healers Association, https://www.soundhealersassociation.org
Gaynor, Mitchell. *The Healing Power of Sound*. Boston: Shambhala, 2002.
Goldman, Jonathan. *The 7 Secrets of Sound Healing*. Carlsbad, CA: Hay House, 2017.

Spirituality

Myss, Caroline. *Anatomy of the Spirit.* New York: Harmony Books, 1996/2017.

Weiss, Brian. *Messages from the Masters.* New York: Warner Books, 2000.

Williamson, Marianne. *A Return to Love.* New York: Harper Perennial, 1992/1996.

Tai Chi

American Tai Chi and Qigong Association, http://www.americantaichi.org

Ubuntu Philosophy

BookAuthority, "100 Best Ubuntu Books of All Time," https://bookauthority .org/books/best-ubuntu-books

Institute for Humane Studies at George Mason University, https://theihs.org /blog/ubuntu-for-everyday

Mathabane, Mark. *The Lessons of Ubuntu: How an African Philosophy Can Inspire Racial Healing in America.* New York: Skyhorse Publishing, 2018.

Ngomane, Mungi. *Everyday Ubuntu: Living Better Together, the African Way.* New York: Harper Design, 2019.

Richards, Shola. *Go Together: How the Concept of Ubuntu Will Change How You Live, Work and Lead.* New York: Sterling Ethos, 2018.

Vegetarian/Vegan Lifestyle*

HappyCow, https://www.happycow.net

One Green Planet, https://www.onegreenplanet.org

Vegetarian Resource Group, https://www.vrg.org

VegSource, https://vegsource.com

Andersen, Kip, and Keegan Kuhn, dirs. *What the Health.* Film. 2017. Santa Rosa, CA: A.U.M. Films & Media. https://www.whatthehealthfilm.com.

Colquhoun, James, and Carlo Ledesma, dirs. *Food Matters.* Film. 2008. Mooloolaba, Queensland, Australia: Permacology Productions. https://www.foodmatters.com/films.

Delforce, Chris, dir. *Dominion.* Film. 2018. https://www.dominionmovement .com.

---

*   See also "Cookbooks" on p. 202 and "Healthy Lifestyle and Diets" on pp. 203–4.

Fulkerson, Lee, dir. *Forks Over Knives*. Film. 2011. Newtown, PA: Virgil Films and Entertainment. https://www.forksoverknives.com/the-film.

Garcia, Deborah Koons, dir. *The Future of Food*. Film. 2004. Burbank, CA: Cinema Libre Studio. https://www.thefutureoffood.com.

Kenner, Robert, dir. *Food Inc*. Film. 2008; Los Angeles: Participant Media. https://robertkennerfilms.com/food_inc.php.

Linklater, Richard, dir. *Fast Food Nation*. Film. 2006. Los Angeles: Fox Searchlight. https://www.searchlightpictures.com/fastfoodnation.

Monson, Shaun, dir. *Earthlings*. 2005. Film. Malibu, CA: Nation Earth. http://www.nationearth.com.

Psihoyos, Louie, dir. *The Game Changers*. Film. 2018. https://gamechangers movie.com.

Wolfson, Marisa Miller, dir. *Vegucated*. Film. 2011. https://vegucated.com/film.

Yoga

American Yoga Association, http://www.americanyogaassociation.net

Yoga Alliance, https://www.yogaalliance.org

Brown, Christina. *The Yoga Bible: The Definitive Guide to Yoga Postures*. Cincinnati, OH: Walking Stick Press, 2003.

Iyengar, B. K. S. *Light on Yoga: The Bible of Modern Yoga*. New York: Schocken Books, 1966/1979.

Stiles, Tara. *Strala Yoga: Be Strong, Focused & Ridiculously Happy from the Inside Out*. Carlsbad, CA: Hay House, 2016.

Index

Page references given in *italics* indicate illustrations or material contained in their captions. Page references followed by an italicized *t*. indicate tables.

About the Author

Jovanka Ciares is an Afro-Latina former entertainment executive turned executive wellness coach, integrative herbalist, nutrition educator, and author. She is the founder and CEO of Solana, an herbal supplement company, and the creator of the education initiative #ReclaimingWellness, which offers education to BIPOC communities on the power of herbal medicine and plant-based living for their healing journey. Born and raised in Puerto Rico, Jovanka now lives in Los Angeles with her partner and her rescue cat King Buddy Kitty.

To extend your wellness journey beyond this book, visit www.reclaimingwellnessbook.com. You can access free bonus resources, including e-courses and information about the author's upcoming speaking and workshop schedule.

For her free and paid courses, visit www.jovankaciares.com /reclaiming-wellness.

And to follow the author on social media, visit these links:

Instagram: www.instagram.com/jovankaciares
Facebook: www.facebook.com/jovankaciares
YouTube: www.youtube.com/user/jovankaciares